# Honor Thy Mother

*Caring for a Loved One Diagnosed with Alzheimer's*

Sheree May

ISBN 979-8-88616-039-0 (paperback)
ISBN 979-8-88616-040-6 (digital)



Christian Faith Publishing
832 Park Avenue
Meadville, PA 16335
www.christianfaithpublishing.com

Printed in the United States of America

# Acknowledgments

My sincere appreciation and gratitude to the following:

- First and foremost, my Lord and Savior Jesus Christ. He has blessed my life and provided the guidance, discipline, and insight needed to make this story possible to share with the world!
- Debra Williams, my supportive sister who is my mentor and best friend. Your contribution to the content in this book is priceless. Your advice and knowledge are always highly valued.
- Christie Eve Dale, my loving daughter who's in charge of Mom's hygiene. I congratulate you on all your accomplishments. You have played such a big role in this family and this story. I've watched you grow into such a God-fearing, God-loving woman. I love you so much!
- Everyone at church on the Rock in St. Peters, Missouri. Your gracious and welcoming spirit touched my heart. Your sharing and caring attitude gave me hope.
- My brothers Willie James Williams Jr and Kevin Eubanks for always checking in to see how their mother is doing.
- My aunt Joan Lofton, who would take us to church when we were very young. Your faith has brought light into so many young hearts. Thanks for calling every day to see how your sister is doing. You have been my inspiration and my light!
- My granddaughter, Keyonna Sheree Williams, who was the inspiration behind the design of the book cover.

- My grandsons Kenneth Carter III and Kendrick Carter who always believed in me.
- My very good friend Georgia Latimer who I truly believed was sent to me by God. Your faith, your prayers, and your positive attitude always made me smile. You are truly a covenant friend.
- My new sister by another mother, Anne Mabry, who is an ordained minister. I will always remember your encouraging words of great wisdom. You are such an amazing and accomplished woman and mother. You are godsent to my sister. We are blessed to have you in our lives.
- Marie Lewis, senior literary agent, whom I know God sent to provide advice and guidance. I am blessed to have someone in my corner who has lived in my shoes. Your experience, knowledge, and professionalism will be my guiding light!
- And last but certainly not least, my mother, Helen Kennebrew. You have inspired me since birth. You have taught me how to love, how to be selfless, and how to forgive. It is such a blessing to see you hug your great, great grandchildren! I am blessed to be in the presence of such a loving mother whom I will always adore and honor!

# Foreword

I have been my mother's caregiver for approximately nine years. Throughout those years, I developed a close relationship with God. I rely on his guidance when I must make tough decisions.

My sister and I took on specific roles in caring for our mother who was diagnosed with Alzheimer's. Her role focused on improving Mom's nutrition. My role focused on keeping Mom's spirits up.

Like a person who childproofs his or her home when expecting a new arrival, I have created an indelible or "forget-proof" environment for my mother. I planted items around the home that would hopefully bring the same joy today that they brought to Mom yesterday. Her photo album from her sixty-fifth birthday party sits on the dining room table. Her customized calendar with a picture of her mother and her seven sisters sits on top of the mantle in the family room. I found recordings of her favorite television shows and movies like *The Carol Burnett Show, I Love Lucy, Diff'rent Strokes, The Golden Girls, Cinderella, Happy Feet*, and others, which we watch together.

I remember how much my mom loved to travel. I still plan small trips to take her on with my daughter and sister.

I have had to make important choices as my mom's caregiver—choices that people didn't agree with. Those choices made me feel as if my life was going in circles, yet I kept the faith, and the end results always brought things into perspective.

As a caregiver, I went from being self-centered to being selfless. I hope my story will paint a picture of God's amazing work through me as my mom's caregiver. I hope my actions, including my mistakes, will help others make better decisions in the care of their loved ones. Thank you for reading my story!

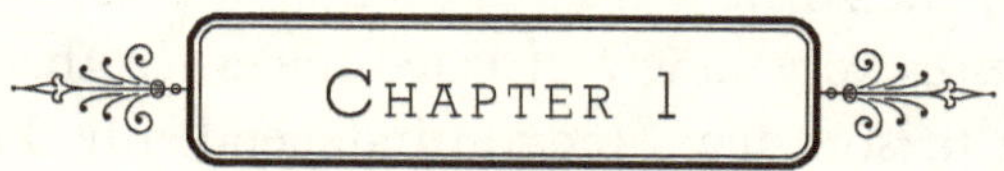



# CHAPTER 1

# Mom's Kodak Memories

I remember the surprise birthday party we gave Mom when she turned sixty-five years old. It was seventeen years ago.

I remember so well because there were over 400 pictures taken during the party. My sister had placed a disposable camera on each table for guests to use. It was one enormous "Kodak moment"!

Today, my mom still pulls out her photo album filled with photos of her children, sisters, nieces, nephews, and friends dancing at her party. I watch her as she flips through pages and pages of pictures. I ask her whom does she recognize at the party. The list grows shorter and shorter each time.

Mom is eighty-two years old. She was diagnosed with Alzheimer's several years ago. Her memory has been gradually slipping away for the past eight years. She was diagnosed in 2014. Today is January 2022. My sister and I took on specific roles in caring for our mom. My sister has studied nutrition most of her life. She is in control of Mom's nutrition.

I am focused on Mom's quality of life. I work to keep her spirits up. I have always been blessed with a good memory. I am sixty-three years old and can remember events from when I was in the third grade. I remember the stories my mom told me about her childhood. I now tell them to her exactly how she told them to me. I remember Mom's favorite television shows that made her laugh. I have found and recorded them so we can laugh together when we watch them.

I remember how Mom loved the smell of gingerbread that her mom used to bake for Christmas. Every holiday, there would be gingerbread baking in the oven.

I read on the Alzheimer's Association website that the disease usually progresses very slowly in three stages. In the early stage of Alzheimer's, a person may function independently. He or she may still drive, work, and be part of social activities. Common difficulties include coming up with the right word or name, remembering names when introduced to new people, having difficulty performing tasks in social or work settings, forgetting material that was just read, losing or misplacing a valuable object, and experiencing increased trouble with planning or organizing. Mom was in this stage when I started taking her on cruises during her retirement.

Middle-stage Alzheimer's is said to be the longest stage. It can last for many years. Here, the symptoms are more pronounced. The person may confuse words, get frustrated or angry, and act in unexpected ways such as refusing to bathe. Symptoms, which vary from person to person, include being forgetful of events or personal history, feeling moody or withdrawn, especially in socially or mentally challenging situations, being unable to recall information about themselves like their address or telephone number, experiencing confusion about where they are or what day it is, requiring help choosing proper clothing for the season or the occasion, having trouble controlling their bladder or bowels, experiencing changes in sleep patterns, such as sleeping during the day and becoming restless at night, showing an increased tendency to wander and become lost, and demonstrating personality and behavioral changes including suspiciousness and delusions or compulsive, repetitive behavior like hand-wringing or tissue shredding. My mom has been showing all these symptoms for a couple of years. It was more noticeable when we moved to Colorado Springs in May 2020. I probably noticed more because I had less distraction there.

The late stage is the final stage. Here, individuals lose the ability to respond to their environment, to carry on a conversation and, eventually, to control movement. They may still say words or phrases, but communicating pain becomes difficult. The symptoms during the late stage include requiring around-the-clock assistance with daily personal care; losing awareness of recent experiences as well as of their surroundings; experiencing changes in physical abilities, including walking, sitting, and eventually swallowing; having difficulty communicating; and becoming vulnerable to infections, especially pneumonia. I feel so grateful that Mom can still walk, although she complains about her hips hurting. She is starting to show signs of difficulty communicating pain. When my daughter tells her she is going to take her to the doctor, Mom refuses to go. She tells her there is nothing wrong with her and that she feels perfectly fine. Thirty minutes later, Mom says her back and hips are killing her, and she needs to get it checked out. Ten minutes later, her back and hips are fine, but her knees and feet are hurting so bad that she may need a wheelchair soon.

Alzheimer's disease tends to develop slowly and gradually worsen over several years. Eventually, Alzheimer's disease affects most areas of your brain. Memory, thinking, judgment, language, problem-solving, personality, and movement can all be affected by the disease.

I am the oldest of four living siblings. My sister, Debra Williams, is one year younger. I have two younger brothers—Willie Williams Jr and Kevin Eubanks. I have lived with Mom most of my life. I was the last to leave home, and when Mom's husband died, she came to live with me.

Our closeness has given me the opportunity to store a lifetime of memories. I also have firsthand knowledge of all the things my mom enjoys in life. I know what makes her smile. I know what makes her sad. I know what music she likes to listen to and the food she likes to eat.

I remember when my mom told me that her mother had thrown her a surprise party for her thirtieth birthday. It was during the late '60s. Mom was the seventh child of ten girls. My mom was a divorced mother of four children. I was the oldest and in the fourth grade.

A few months before Mom's thirtieth birthday, she met her prince charming—my new stepdad. His name was Jacob Eubanks.

Everyone called him Jake. My mom met him when she was visiting Grandma in the hospital. Jake was in a room down the hall.

One day, my mom came to visit her mother, and Jake was sitting in Grandma's room talking to her. They started a conversation, and the rest is history.

Jake was tall, dark, and handsome. He also had the personality to match his looks—very charming! My grandma was very pleased when my mom started dating Jake. The whole family was pleased. He had warmed his way into everyone's heart. I even took a liking to him immediately, and I was not easily swayed. I could always sense good in a person. Jake was good, loving, and kind. He helped Grandma plan Mom's surprise party.

Grandma had the party at the Cutrate. It was a tavern across from Hunter's Meat Packing Plant. My mom was one of the first black women to get hired at the plant. She was a pork boner. It was hard work. She always came home covered in blood. It was impossible to wash hog's blood from the white frocks she wore to work.

I remember watching my mom get dressed for work. She would put on many layers of clothes. She said she worked inside a freezer. The room had to be cold to keep the meat from thawing. Mom used sharp knives to take the bone out of half-frozen hams. One frozen ham weighed more than I did. It was very dangerous work. The knife could easily slip and take off a finger. Many people walked away from the plant with missing parts.

Men who worked at the plant didn't think women belonged there. They weren't receptive to women coming in to do a "man's job". The work environment became hostile, especially to young black women like my mom. I remember her telling me that frozen hams were being flung onto the conveyor belt near her. One frozen ham weighed at least twenty pounds. If one of those hams hit my mom, it could put her in the hospital. She said that no man was going to prevent her from putting food on the table for her kids. Mom became like a bear protecting her cubs. My mom had a big bark that made those bullies back off.

Have you ever heard of the Black Panthers?

The Black Panthers was a political party founded in Oakland, California, in 1966 by Huey Newton and Bobby Seale. The group, which wore black berets and black leather jackets, challenged police brutality against African American communities. It is said that there were roughly 2000 members in which some were involved in deadly shootouts. Although the Black Panthers were considered a gang by many, they were part of a larger Black Power movement, which focused on Black pride, community control, and equality in the workplace.

J. Edgar Hoover, the first FBI Director, called the Black Panthers "one of the greatest threats to the nation's internal security."

Educator and activist Angela Davis joined the Black Panthers. She was known for her involvement in feminism, race, and the prison system in the United States.

We were the Davis family. My mom told me that Grandma was getting a lot of phone calls from California during the mid-'60s. Grandma's name is Mary Davis. I don't know if Mom believed that Angela Davis was a relative or not. All I know is that if anyone thought you were affiliated with the Panthers during the late '60s, they would immediately back off.

I just know that, that very same week, those men who had been mean to my mom started asking her if they could sharpen her knives for her. Sharp knives made boning the hams much easier. That's all I'm saying.

Grandma invited all the workers at the plant and the residents of Goose Hill to my mom's birthday party. Most of them came and bought a round of drinks for everyone. The neighbors on Goose Hill heard about the free drinks and free food and came to wish Mom a happy birthday. Everyone took turns playing music on the jukebox. I imagine Mom being treated like the "godfather," or shall I say god-mother on that day. My mom said that she drank so much Crown Royal and 7 Up that she didn't remember much of what happened at her party.

The following day, Mom woke up with a hangover. I remember Jake taking care of her. He happily took on the role of "Mr. Mom." That wasn't easy for any man to do in those days. The men were looked on as the "breadwinner" of the family. My mom put on the hard hat, and Jake put on the apron. It was the perfect match. I was so happy that my stepdad started cooking our meals because he was the better cook.

There were lots of barbecues in the late '60s and early '70s. My mom always brought a box of ribs from her job. Our family became some of the biggest carnivores. It seemed like every month we were having a picnic and eating barbecue ribs.

One day, I noticed that my stepdad seemed unusually happy. He took my two siblings and me on a drive to share with us what he called "good news." He said that there was going to be a new addition to the family. Mom was going to have a baby. We were going to have a new sister or brother. The three of us were sitting in the back seat of the car. We looked at each other. There was no expression of joy on our little faces. I couldn't understand why Mom would even want another baby.

I remember hearing horror stories of my mom giving birth. My mom had a lot of difficulty with four of her childbirths. Mom gave birth to six children, three were breech births. Mom's first born was my brother, Demetrius. He was born with birth defects. He died when I was twelve years old. I didn't get to know him because he lived at a medical facility in Lincoln, Illinois. I was the second child. My sister came a year after me. Mom said she tried to come out arm first. Mom's fourth child was a girl. She tried to come out feet first. The doctors turned her around. My mom said that when she was born, she saw her daughter's head drop and knew she had died right there in the delivery room. My mom slipped into a coma after she saw her daughter's little head drop. She could hear the doctors telling her mom that she would be dead by morning. My grandmother just held mom's hand and started praying. She could feel her mom's tears fall on her hand. My mom said she had left her body and was floating on the ceiling looking down at everything that was happening. Up there on the ceiling, she began asking God to spare her life so she could raise her children. She didn't want anyone else raising her children. Hours later, my mom said she woke up and told Grandma that she was so hungry she could eat a hog and its baby pigs. If that wasn't a miracle, then I don't know what is.

One year later, Mom gave birth to my brother. He tried to come out butt first. Again, the doctors had to go in and rearrange the baby. Mom was never put to sleep during these deliveries. I don't understand why she didn't ask to have her tubes tied after the third child. It bewilders me how she still wanted to have ten children as Grandma did.

Eight years later, in 1972, my youngest brother was born. It was the first delivery that my mom was given a sedative. My stepdad did not live long after the birth of his only child. He didn't get a chance to watch his son grow up. Mom once again became a single mom.

When Hunter's Packing Company closed on Goose Hill, my mom went to nursing school. She became a CNA and started working in a nursing home. It was a different kind of hard work. She enjoyed caring for her patients, and they adored her.

My sister and I gave Mom a surprise party on March 3, 2004, the day Mom turned sixty-five years old. Some of her coworkers attended the party. Many people at the party talked about how my mom had impacted their life. Everyone there had a story about how Mom took care of them or their loved ones.

I remember hearing the story about when my mom was around nine years old. She would go to work with her mom who was sickly. Grandma worked at the stockyards cleaning offices.

One day, Granddad was taking all the girls out to dinner. Grandma had to go to work on that day. Everyone left the house together. Grandma headed in one direction, and Granddad headed with the girls in the opposite direction. Mom was one of those girls. Suddenly, my mom stopped walking with Granddad, turned around, and started running in Grandma's direction. She told her dad she was going to go help her mom clean offices. She started walking with Grandma, then suddenly stopped and started running back in Granddad's direction because her little stomach was growling. Mom continually ran back and forth between her parents several times in trying to decide. The neighbors on Goose Hill were sitting on the porch watching and wondering what was wrong with that little girl.

Mom finally settled on staying with her mom and yelled back at her dad to please bring her a hamburger home from the restaurant. Mom was hungry that day, but she didn't let her hunger stop her from looking after her mom.

Mom's caring heart continues today. She has taken her calling as a caregiver to a whole new level. Each of mom's sisters stood up at her party and thanked her for the way she took care of their mother all her life. That night, her sisters showed their gratitude.

One grateful son-in-law talked about how his mother-in-law took a leave of absence from work to come help him care for his wife. She couldn't walk, wash herself, or turn over in bed. After being in a physical rehab unit at Jewish Hospital for over a month, the doctors sent her home in a wheelchair. The doctors had done all they could. The son-in-law needed to go to work but couldn't leave his wife home alone. His mother-in-law came every day to cook, clean, and wash his wife. I was that wife.

I remember the care I received during that painful time in my life. My mom could soothe my pain when doctors and nurses couldn't. Her presence was like therapy. It felt like my spirit was purified or cleansed by my mom's sponge baths. I looked forward to my mom's visits. She never had to say a word because her actions did all the talking.

One grateful granddaughter named Eve talked about what her grandma did for her when she fell and broke both of her arms. Eve said that her grandma is the reason she has a high school diploma. She was in the twelfth grade when both of her arms were in casts. She said her grandma called and talked to her principal and teachers. She then went and got her schoolbooks and homework for her. She even fed and washed her. Eve said she would not have graduated that year if it wasn't for her grandma.

A grateful niece talked about how her aunt Helen cared for both her sister and her mother when they were diagnosed with cancer. She said that every time she called, her aunt dropped whatever she was doing and came. She remembered seeing her sick sister sitting up in bed, eating white rice and beef liver cooked by her aunt Helen. It was her favorite dish.

Mom's boss at River Bluff Nursing Home wrote a letter that read:

> Over 2,000 years ago, God blessed us with the precious gift of his son who died on Calvary for all our sins. Being the gracious and just Father, he gave to this world Helen Kennebrew who, for 65 years, has labored and toiled in the vineyards of life, giving and helping everyone that has ever crossed her path. This precious jewel of God has been a beacon of light for all that has known her. A wonderful mother, grandmother, sister, and most of all a great friend who will go the extra mile to make sure all is well on the home front of life. She is always there to lend an ear whenever one is needed. Always there to help you when you are down on your luck. Always there giving 110% of herself no matter what the task may be. Helen, my friend, you are a diamond in the rough. And God is molding you into something so brilliant and wonderful. We, the staff of the River Bluff Nursing and Rehabilitation Center, would like to take this time to thank you for 18 years of service, 18 years of faithfulness, and 18 years of sharing your love with each and every one of us. May God continue to bless you and may he keep you in perfect peace.

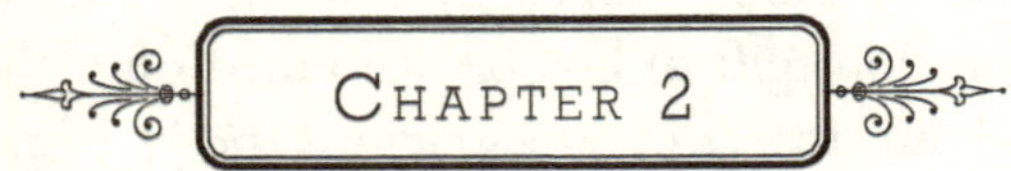

CHAPTER 2

# Mother's Day Cruises

The date was May 9, 2013.

The time was 5:00 a.m.

My alarm clock started to sing.

I rushed to Mom's room to wake her.

We got dressed, packed the car, and left St. Louis heading toward New Orleans.

Nine years after Mom's sixty-fifth birthday, I went from planning her surprise birthday parties to planning her surprise cruises. I took my mom on her first cruise to Cozumel, Mexico. She was seventy-four years old. It was her Mother's Day Gift from me. It was also the first of many cruises to come.

What made this trip so special was that we all were experiencing cruising together for the first time. There were five of us—my mom and I, my daughter and her boyfriend, and my granddaughter.

I remember looking at the expression on everyone's face when we laid eyes on a cruise ship for the first time. Although it was one of the smallest in Carnival's fleet, it was gigantic to us. We all felt like we walked onto a small resort on the ocean.

I had booked a grand suite. I wanted my mom to be comfortable just in case she gets motion sickness. I wanted to make sure she had a nice cabin to lounge in. Little did I know at the time that my mom would hardly be in the cabin. There was so much to do and see on the ship.

We headed straight to the buffet the moment we got on the ship. The large selection of food was overwhelming. Next, we sat out by the pool with a drink and watched people dance as the ship left the dock.

Our days at sea began with eating, followed by going to a game show, then shopping before lunch. After lunch, we would relax by the pool and read a book. Later, we would attend a dance class followed by a live comedy show. Evenings were just as busy. We would enjoy a disco before dinner. Dinner was always followed by a Broadway show. Our day always ended with a comedy show and late-night ice cream.

My favorite part of the cruise was having dinner in the main dining room. The room had white tablecloths and sparkling chandeliers. The waiters pulled our chairs out for us and laid napkins in our lap. I felt like royalty every time I went to dinner. I even found delight in watching my mom enjoy eating salmon, her favorite dish.

We sat at a table with two other families. The first family was a mother and her daughter. The daughter had brought her mom on a cruise as a Mother's Day gift. The second family was a married couple with two college-aged children. Everyone introduced themselves. The family of four were veteran cruisers. Everyone was there to celebrate Mother's Day.

The second night at dinner, everyone talked about what they had planned when we dock in Cozumel the following day. The mother and daughter were going zip-lining. The family of four was going to visit the Mayan Ruins. My family and I hadn't booked any shore excursions. We were just going to walk around and check out the little shops around the dock.

I enjoyed listening to the veteran cruisers talk throughout dinner about all the places they had traveled to. We just sat back and let them take us to beautiful faraway places every night. Some of those places I couldn't wait to take my mom to. Cruising was the beginning of something special, at least I thought at the time. Little did I know it would change soon.

The date was March 2014

The time was 5:00 a.m.

My alarm clock started to sing.

I rushed to Mom's room to wake her.

We got dressed, packed the van, and left St. Louis heading towards New Orleans for our second cruise.

We were going on a seven-day cruise to Jamaica. We rented a van this time because my sister and Mom's best friend joined us. When we arrived at the dock, Mom's friend was afraid to go up the gangway to board the ship. I began to worry because we couldn't leave her behind. My sister took her hand gently and guided her up the gangway while talking to her in a calm voice. I've never seen my sister being patient with anyone. It was fascinating to watch. It took time, but she got her on the ship.

This was a much bigger and newer ship than the one we went on for our first cruise. I was so happy that my sister joined us on this cruise. We went to a '60s disco party on the ship, and she danced with Mom. It was a joy to watch. My mom moved as if she was dancing on air. It has been a long time since I saw her having such a good time. Her energy was at an all-time high. I told my sister I had never seen Mom move with such grace before. I thought cruising had brought life back into our mom.

Mom had retired several years ago. She came to live with me after her third husband died. It happened only a couple of years after her sixty-fifth birthday. She started assisting me with my part-time eBay business. I would buy bundles of jewelry, and she would sort through and organize the jewelry for me so I could list the pieces online. She ended up keeping most of the jewelry which she now wears on the cruises. I love watching her dress up for dinner on the ship.

The following day, my sister discovered what became our favorite part of the ship—the serenity deck. This area of the ship was exclusive for adults twenty-one years and older. It became Mom's and my favorite hangout. The deck overlooked the pool where everyone on the ship hung out. It was quiet and peaceful where we sat. There were chaise lounges, sofas, hammocks, a hot tub, and a bar. It became Mom's and my little paradise on the ship. It sat three stories above the main pool. We could look down at the entrance to the buffet. We watched people come and go from the buffet carrying plates loaded with food. We studied parents struggling to get their children out of the pool. We read books, flipped through magazines, and talked.

I asked Mom if she was enjoying being retired. She said thanks to me, she feels like she has died and gone to heaven. Mom said that if she died today and came back tomorrow, she wanted her same children.

I loved having Mom live with me. We have always been close. She helped raise my daughter Eve when I went into the military at nineteen years old. Eve stayed with my mom when my marriage to her dad failed. My mom had always been there for me. It was my time to be there for her.

The ship docked in Jamaica on day three of our second cruise. We were getting ready to leave the ship to visit Jamaica. I noticed that Mom was sitting on the side of the bed. She seemed upset. I asked her if anything was wrong. She told me that someone had taken her red blouse out of her luggage. I looked in the closet and drawers for her blouse. I then asked if she was sure she had packed it. She said she was sure. I wanted to believe her, but I had given my mom two white blouses to pack for me, and they weren't in the luggage when we arrived on the ship. I picked up another blouse for her to wear that I thought would go very well with her pants. I then told her when we returned to the ship that I would help her find her red blouse. We then headed out to explore Jamaica.

A dark-skinned man wearing a huge nappy afro wig approached us. He asked if we needed a tour guide. We immediately said no and walked quickly away from him. He was scary-looking. A few minutes later, we were still standing around wondering what we should do. We wanted a driver to take us around. There was a lady who seemed in charge at the dock. She was assigning drivers to tourists as they walked off the ship. We told her we wanted someone to drive us to the beach. She motioned for a driver who ended up being the man we had recently run from. Hesitantly, we agreed to let him take us to the beach. I thought that if the ship staff was okay with him, then we should be safe.

We all got into his van, and as he started to drive, he asked if this was our first time in Jamaica. We answered yes. He then told us that we shouldn't waste our time going to the beach when there were so many other places we should see. He offered to take us to a new pier that had just opened. He said it was much better than the one our ship had docked at. Since he lived in Jamaica, I thought he knew where we should go better than we did. We took his advice.

I was sitting in the front seat looking horrified as the driver sped through town. He swerved around goats and chickens. I had never ridden in a car with anyone who drove so fast. I searched for a speed limit sign and couldn't find one. I wanted to close my eyes, but I was too scared not to see what was happening. I sat in silence, hoping that we would reach our destination in one piece. We did!

The driver was right. The pier was beautiful. There was also a festival taking place across from the pier. We got to mingle with lots of locals. We took lots of pictures. The driver was very friendly. He had a constable get us a golf cart to ride in because my mom and I walked with a cane. He was a gentleman. He helped Mom into the golf cart. He also went and bought two bottles of cold water for Mom and me. It was very hot in Jamaica. The scary-looking, wild driver turned out to be a gentle saint.

The date was June 2014.

The time was 6:00 a.m.

My alarm clock started to sing.

I rushed to Mom's room to wake her.

We got dressed, packed the car, and headed to the airport.

We were taking the plane to Seattle. There we would board the ship to Alaska.

This was my mom's first time on a plane. She was not receptive to walking through the metal detectors. She didn't like having her luggage searched. Mom was really upset when airport security took her large bottles of mouth wash and lotion. She asked if he was going to pay her for them. I never heard my mom use profanity as she did at the airport.

This trip was different from the previous two cruises. Mom kept saying this would be her last trip. My daughter kept saying she was never going to take my mom anywhere ever again.

Mom was never happy throughout the trip to Alaska. I remember my mom's first reaction when I told her that I was taking her to Alaska. She said why. I told her because I always wanted to go to Alaska. Again, she asked why. I said I thought it was one of the most beautiful, untamed places on earth. I don't think anyone was as excited as I was to be going to Alaska.

When we arrived in our cabin to unpack, I was surprised to find our luggage didn't have one warm item of clothing. All the clothing I had laid out to pack was never packed. I had to go to the shop on the ship to buy clothes for Mom and me. I asked my mom why she didn't pack the clothes I had put out for her to pack. She told me that I never gave her any clothes to pack. It was then I started to realize that something was not right with Mom. I didn't want to spoil our vacation, so I put my concerns aside and tried to enjoy Alaska.

The ship took us through the Tracy Arm fjord. I couldn't believe how cold it was in Alaska in June. We all had our coats on as we cruised through the fjord passing through glaciers. There were giant chunks of ice floating in the ocean. I was hoping to see a whale but didn't. The ship docked the next day in Skagway. I felt as if I had traveled back in time. I decided to splurge on a shore excursion for the first time. I booked the White Pass Yukon train ride.

It was the best ride of my life. Mom and I sat together on the train. I sat by the window. The train started moving slowly. The train's whistle blew. The steel wheels started squealing as the train crawled alongside one of the most popular trails in history, the Yukon trail.

I took a train ride that crept through the wilds of mother nature and ascended into the clouds. The train crawled through Alaska's rough exterior. We traveled along the iconic trail where it is said that 3000 horses fell over the cliff. How could something so beautiful be so deadly?

I glanced over at the narrow Yukon trail and couldn't believe the risk people would take in search of gold. I wondered why someone would rather be dead than poor.

We passed gigantic waterfalls and crossed over mile-deep ravines. We rounded cliff-hanging turns of sixteen degrees. As we neared the top, it was like looking down into the abyss. My life took on a whole new meaning. Up there beyond the clouds, only God could keep me on track. I was no longer riding on steel tracks and wood trestles. I put my faith in God. It was a spiritual journey over nature's untamed beauty.

When we arrived back at the ship, I asked my mom how did she like the train ride. She said it was the most expensive nap she had ever taken. Mom never warmed up throughout this trip, figuratively speaking.

The date was April 20, 2015.

The time was 5:30 a.m.

The alarm clock sang.

I rushed into Mom's room to wake her, but she is already up getting dressed.

This would be the cruise of all cruises. I was taking my mom and three of her sisters to a Smokey Robinson concert onboard the ship.

That morning, we took a plane to Florida. There we boarded the ship for a five-day cruise. The concert would take place when we dock in Cozumel, Mexico. Smokey would board the ship there to perform that evening. Everyone seemed excited. Aunt Joanie, mom's youngest sister, kept thinking that she was going to a Lionel Richie concert. She probably was trying to give me a hint.

My aunts were having a good time on the ship. They hung out at the piano bar listening to the tunes of the '60s. They went to comedy shows. There Aunt Joanie's laughter was funnier than the jokes.

I enjoyed dinner in the main dining room with Mom and my aunts. We met another couple at the table. There was great food, great conversation, and lots of laughter. Everyone seemed to be having a good time! Mom seemed to be having a good time one minute and crying the next.

Mom's condition seemed to be escalating during each vacation. She complained about the crowd on the ship. She complained about the cold. She complained about the noise. She complained about too much walking. Yet Mom turned down everything we offered to help improve her situation. She didn't want to use my motorized scooter which I take on every cruise. She said she may run into people if she drove the scooter. She said it was too many people on the ship for her to maneuver. Mom's complaining never ceased. I hoped the concert would put her in a better mood.

The concert took place on the third night of the cruise. We had front row seats, a private photo shoot with the singer, and free drinks during the performance. The look on my mother and aunts' faces that evening was priceless. I had never felt so much joy in watching how my aunts were enjoying themselves at the concert. They knew how to have a good time. It was the sparkle in their eyes that made me feel that all my hard work in planning this trip had paid off. My aunts were having fun and it showed.

We sat in the third row from the stage. Smokey sang and danced his way into our hearts. My aunts knew the words to all his songs. I didn't want the night to end.

The next day following the concert, Mom complained that a lot of her personal items were missing from the cabin. She claimed that someone had taken a necklace. I have never seen Mom wearing a necklace, yet I didn't dispute her. I offered to help her look for the missing jewelry. I even offered to take her to the jewelry store on the ship to find a nice necklace to replace the one that was missing. She wanted that necklace because she said it belonged to her mother. I asked Mom to describe how the necklace looked so I can search for it. She described it, and it sounded exactly like the one she and I had been admiring earlier in one of the shops on the ship. I went and purchased that exact necklace and put it under her pillow that evening. Mom found the necklace under her pillow that evening. She thought the cabin steward had snuck it back in to keep from getting fired. I didn't say anything about it.

The last night of the cruise, my frustration with how my mom had been behaving got the best of me. It was during dinner. We were all getting up from the table deciding how we wanted to spend our last night. When I stood up from the table, my mom was standing next to me. She asked me for the fourth time in the last five minutes if I was going to the cabin to go to bed because that's what she wanted to do. I had just told her I was going to a farewell party on the Lido deck with my sister. I told her that she should spend some time with her sisters who were going to the piano bar. My mom didn't want to do that. I started yelling at her about how she had made this vacation miserable for everyone. I told her that I was tired of wasting my money on her because she didn't know how to appreciate anything. I called her selfish and inconsiderate. Mom started to cry. I immediately begged for forgiveness. I had never spoken to my mom like that before. I had never raised my voice at my mom. I saw myself as the worse daughter ever. I asked for God's help that last night on the ship.

> Dear Lord, I lost my way, please find me before I'm gone forever.
> Here, spirits are low; tempers are high. No mercy whatsoever!
> Not only have I abused, betrayed, rejected— my mother's needs I have neglected.
> My eyes were closed, my ears clogged—my heart was cold!
> I plead for your mercy! I pray for my soul!
> Amen.

A good daughter would not take her mom to places that made her uncomfortable. A caring daughter would see that her mom is miserable on cruises. The ships were always cold. Her things always came up missing. The ships were too big and required too much walking. There were too many people and too much noise. She just wanted to stay home. Mom's cruising days had come to an end.

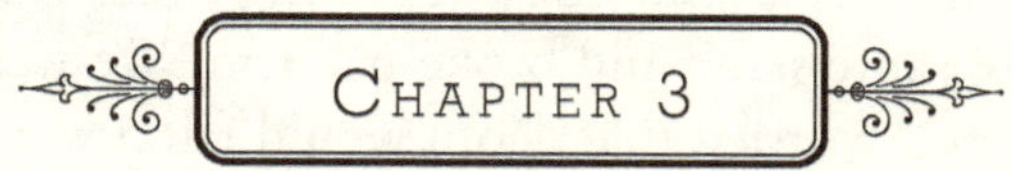

# CHAPTER 3

# Seven Moves in Five Years

A loud knock at my bedroom door woke me up.

I looked over at my phone. It was 5:00 a.m.

The door opened, and my mom peeped through it.

Mom told me that she had packed up her room and was ready to leave. She asked what time we are leaving.

I replied by asking, "Where are we going?"

My mom, looking puzzled, asked, "Aren't we going home?"

I told her that we were home.

Mom then asked, "Who lives here?"

I told her that we did.

She asked, "How long have we been living here?"

I told her it's been a couple of years.

She said that she didn't know that we were living here. She then closed my door and went back to her room.

A half hour later, Mom opened my door and asked what time we are leaving.

Could this have been the outcome of our moving seven times in the last five years?

The first big move happened seven years ago. After twenty-five years of living in the same place, I told my husband, David, it was time for us to move. We lived in a condo with lots of stairs. There were thirty-two steps to our front door. Once inside, there were twenty-one steps up to our bedroom. We had so many memories here. David and I were married in our home twenty-five years ago. There were great and not-so-great memories.

My stepdad fell down the steps outside and busted both of his knees. He was in the hospital for a very long time. Not long after, I fell down those same stairs and broke my arm. We were getting too old for the stairs. I worried that Mom would fall down the stairs one day. That thought haunted me constantly.

Mom came to live with us when my stepdad died. She was approaching her seventies. I worried every time she went up and down the stairs. She would always try to console me by saying that the stairs were keeping her young. She saw the stairs as her only exercise. I just couldn't take the chance of her falling down those stairs.

The first time I talked to my husband about moving, he said no. We had taken a reverse mortgage on the condo. We only paid condo fees. David loved the idea of no rent and no mortgage. He said he didn't want another mortgage.

My husband had surgery due to an injury at work. It was difficult for him to go up and down the stairs. My mom also started showing signs of dementia. She started going up and down the stairs frequently because she kept forgetting things. I decided to bring up moving again. It seemed like the perfect opportunity. I told my husband that my daughter wanted us to get a place together so she can help with the expenses. David reluctantly agreed.

It took several months for my daughter, Christie, and me to find a place that could accommodate five adults. We wanted three or four bedrooms and at least three bathrooms.

We found a beautiful home for rent on Cousteau. The home had three bedrooms, two baths, and a large kitchen with plenty of pantry and cabinets. The design was an open floor plan with high beam ceilings in the living area. There was also a finished basement which my daughter loved. The only issue was there was no bathroom in the basement. The home was in a perfect location. Two of my mother's sisters lived nearby.

Though everything seemed good, I had problems adjusting to the move.

The first night in the new home, I dreamt that I was trying to get back to the condo, but I couldn't find my way back. I kept getting lost and calling out to my husband for help. I had that dream for several nights. I would always wake up sweating. I tried to convince myself that I had made the right decision to move and that the dreams meant nothing.

The Cousteau rental was in a fabulous neighborhood. It was very quiet. I enjoyed walks with my daughter. My mom and I spent a lot of time on the patio when the grandchildren visited. We loved watching them play in the large fenced-in backyard. They loved to run and jump. I would get exhausted just watching. It was almost the perfect place until we faced one issue—not enough bathrooms.

My mom, husband, and I shared a bathroom. It always seemed like my mom and my husband needed to use the bathroom at the same time. My daughter and I started looking for a home with at least three bathrooms. We moved once our one-year lease ended.

We tried to find a home in the same area but didn't have any luck. We moved about five miles from Cousteau into a house on Fairmount. We signed a two-year lease. The neighborhood seemed like a step-down. However, the home had three bathrooms and enough bedrooms. My daughter loved the basement. It was like a whole new apartment with two bedrooms, a bathroom, and a living room. It was only missing a kitchen.

I noticed a few things about the house after living there a couple of months—the neighbors!

I worked from home and couldn't work on the weekends because that's when my neighbors liked to party. The homes were so close that I could hear their music and conversation. They also had a dog that liked to bark all night. My business began to suffer. I had to endure for two years before I could make another move. I never realized how long it was going to take to find a place to settle in once I had left my condo of twenty-five years. My daughter and I started house hunting three months from when our lease would end.

This time, I found a house twenty miles from Fairmount. The house sat on a private road which attracted me instantly. There was only one neighbor, and their house wasn't close. The house was surrounded by a wooded area. I knew I would be able to work without any issues. My daughter moved into the walkout basement.

I thought I had found the perfect place until the day my husband had to leave the house to go to the doctor. We always took my husband to the doctor in a wheelchair. Well, it was almost impossible to push the wheelchair up the hill to the car from the house.

The home in Blackjack was situated on the side of a hill. We had to walk up the hill to get to the car. It was difficult for my husband, Mom, and me to leave. I knew we couldn't spend a winter in this house. My daughter and I decided to look for a home to buy this time since we now knew all the things we needed to make our living arrangements work.

We expanded our search. I thought it would be great to live near the church I liked to attend. It was in another city. My daughter found a real estate agent to help us. I never had looked at so many homes in my life. We would tour home after home and say either the rooms were too small, or it was missing a family room, or the kitchen was too small, or the neighbors were too close, or the neighborhood was too busy. There was always something. I think we looked at over fifty homes before we found one that we wanted to make an offer on. It was the closest to being perfect. There were two homes we made offers on. The first home was love at first sight. The minute I walked into the house on Pyrenees Drive, I knew this was the home for my family. There were five bedrooms and four bathrooms. There was a living room and a family room. There was a dining room and an eat-in kitchen. The home had hardwood floors. The family room had a woodburning fireplace. The basement was a walkout. There was also a screened-in sunporch that overlooked the nine-hole golf course out back. I had to have this house!

The second home we made an offer on was the one my daughter and her boyfriend liked. It also had five bedrooms and four bathrooms. I wasn't too keen on the area. It was a beautiful home but not like the one on Pyrenees Drive. When we put in both offers, I prayed for the house on Pyrenees Drive.

My daughter rushed into my bedroom to tell me the good news. Our offer was accepted on the second house. It wasn't the house on

Pyrenees Drive. I was happy because my daughter was happy. The house had everything we wanted. I was okay with the outcome.

My daughter and I went to the house during the inspection. The inspector said it was a very nice home. He was only concerned with the foundation in the basement and the roof. He told us that we would need to get a new roof in a couple of years. After the inspection, my daughter requested the owner have a new roof put on and take care of the foundation issue in the basement. The owner didn't accept our request for the new roof. My daughter went over to the house to meet the owner. It had been raining that week. When my daughter went into the basement, there was a flood. The owner said that he would fix the leak in the basement. My daughter and I started to think if this purchase would be a big mistake. The next day, the real estate agent called my daughter to let her know that the home on Pyrenees Drive was back on the market. We immediately saw this as a blessing. We resubmitted our offer, and after some negotiating, the Pyrenees house was ours.

Praise God!

The move into the house on Pyrenees Drive was the fourth move since we left the condo four years ago. There were going to be three more moves within the next year and a half. I hadn't at this point noticed the effects the moves were having on Mom. There could have been issues I was just too busy focusing on what I thought was important at the time.

We invited all our family and friends to our new home to have Thanksgiving dinner with us. My mom was sitting at the table with her four sisters. They were talking about things that happened during their childhood. Everyone was laughing and having a good time. We were all one big happy family that night!

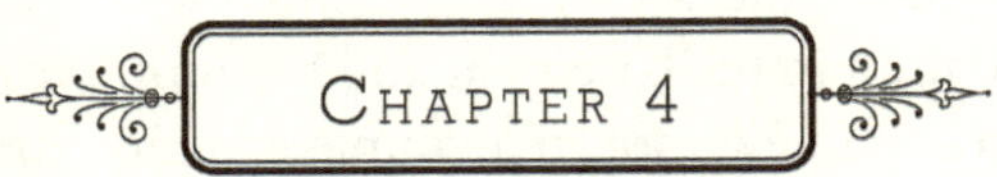

# Mother Rebekah

"My name is Sheree. I am a faithful believer in Jesus Christ. I suffer from anxiety, codependency, Godlike tendencies, and trust issues.

"I came here to Celebrate Recovery to keep an eye on my daughter. She is attending for her gambling addiction. I can't go on her word that she's getting help because she has broken her word too many times.

"I feel, as her mother, it's my duty to make sure she gets the help she needs. We have been to Gambler's Anonymous at least five times. Those visits didn't have any impact or influence on motivating her to stop gambling. So here we are.

"My daughter says that she goes to the casino to relieve stress. It bothers her to be in her home watching the people she loves suffer. Her grandma, who is seventy-nine years old, has dementia. Eve used to be able to talk to her about anything, but now she is unable to. The only thing her grandmother does now is say she is ready to meet her Maker or that she needs to sign herself into a nursing home. She says it every day, sometimes several times a day. Also, my husband, David, Eve's stepfather, is seventy-seven years old and recently had Bariatric surgery. It left him very weak in his legs. He only leaves his recliner to go to the bathroom. My daughter brings his meals to him when she's home. I have put too much on my daughter. I have added so much stress to my daughter's life once I moved in with her. She now lives with two ailing senior citizens and one disabled parent—that's me. I have a muscle weakness disability. I walk with a cane for balance and stability. I am unable to drive a motor vehicle. My daughter has to drive us to our doctor's appointments, dentist appointments, YMCA, and anywhere else we need to go.

"My daughter and I recently purchased a home we both love. It took several years of searching to find such a place with enough space to accommodate five adults. Yet, it's not a loving home. I hope that coming here will help me get closer to God so he can fix my relationship with my daughter.

"Thanks for letting me share."

The topic at my first meeting was about putting the first principle in Celebrate Recovery into action—realizing I'm not God.

"I must accept that I am powerless, and my life is unmanageable."

I have this major tendency to judge people according to how I would act or be. I am so disappointed when my daughter tells me she is going to church, and she ends up at the casino. I think to myself, *What kind of person would lie to their mother? How could she be so deceitful? How could she be my child because I would never do such things?* She needs help. It took a while before I realized that I am powerless to control my daughter's actions. Today's lesson made me aware that all my troubles and heartaches could have been avoided if I had just given it all over to God and trusted in him to make it right. It's a lot easier said than done. I needed to recite the serenity prayer several times a day, starting first thing every morning, 'God, grant me the serenity to accept the things I cannot change, the courage to change the things I can, and the wisdom to know the difference.'

I don't know how my daughter and I happened upon Celebrate Recovery. It was there when I realized I needed just as much, or even maybe more, help than my daughter. I was hooked after attending the first meeting.

I liked the way the meeting was structured. First, we all worship together, then we break into small groups to talk and discuss what's on our minds. The groups are divided first by sex—all males in one group and all females in the other group. Then those groups are broken down by specific issues such as alcohol and drugs, eating disorders, codependency, etc.

I felt good when I left my first meeting at Celebrate Recovery. Everyone there had been very welcoming. There, I could learn how to fix my relationship with God. There, I could spill out my guts, and no one will look at me any different. There, we all were broken, and no one judged. Everyone came to spill, and only God was there to heal.

When my daughter and I returned home from Celebrate Recovery, I asked to borrow her study Bible. I have prayed since I was a child. Many of my aunts took me to church throughout my childhood. I always knew there was a God. I just don't think I ever worked on getting to really know God through his word. I always listened to sermons. I attempted to read the Bible many times throughout my life. I never made it past the book of Genesis. When I opened Celebrate Recovery's Study Bible, it was different. The human stories that surrounded the scriptures kept me intrigued. The testimonials throughout the book gave me hope. I started reading the Bible alone in my bedroom every night at 9:30. I closed the physical door to my room and opened the spiritual door to God.

I was intrigued by the story of Esau and Jacob. That story made me realize how fortunate I was to have a mother who never showed favoritism to any of her children. My sister brought home better grades than I did. My mother never treated me any different, though she offered to get me a tutor. Many people said my sister was prettier than I was. My mother was never one of those people. She treated us like we were twins. She bought me the same beautiful clothes she bought my sister. She styled my hair the same way she styled my sister's. We were twins in her eyes.

Isaac and Rebekah had twin sons. The sons were different. One was a hunter, and the other was a domestic. One would think they would complement each other very well. For example, the differences between my sister and me elevated the level of care we gave our mother. Unfortunately, it wasn't the case for these two brothers. The parents may have been responsible. Isaac favored the oldest son who was a "manly man". Rebekah favored the youngest son who liked to use his wits over physical strength. This caused a feud that led all the way to the birth of Jesus as the story goes:

> Isaac was forty years old when he married Rebekah, daughter of Bethuel, the Aramean from Paddan Aram and sister of Laban the Aramean.
>
> Isaac prayed to the Lord on behalf of his wife because she was childless. The Lord answered his prayer, and his wife Rebekah became pregnant. The babies jostled each other within her, and she said, "Why is this happening to me?" So she went to inquire of the Lord. The Lord said to her, "Two nations are in your womb, and two peoples from within you will be separated: one people will be stronger than the other, and the older will serve the younger."
>
> When the time came for her to give birth, there were twin boys in her womb. The first to come out was red, and his whole body was like a hairy garment, so they named him Esau. After this, his brother came out, with his hand grasping Esau's heel, so he was named Jacob.
>
> The boys grew up, and Esau became a skillful hunter, a man of the open country, while Jacob was content to stay at home among the tents. Isaac, who had a taste for wild game, loved Esau, but Rebekah loved Jacob.

I know how it feels to have a parent show more affection toward your sibling than you. My father, whom I didn't know was actually my stepfather, would always buy my sister toys and not me. He would take her to special events and not me. I was nine years old. It still hurts when I think about it. It was my mom who tried to make up for what my stepfather didn't give me. Her attention and affection sustained me during those trying times. Yet I believed my adult life was affected by the one-sided love I received as a child. I married a man nearly twenty years older than me. I think I was looking for that fatherly affection I hardly received as a child. What I'm saying is that a relationship between a parent and a child could influence how that child lives throughout his entire life!

Back to the story of Esau and Jacob:

> Once when Jacob was cooking some stew, Esau came in from the open country, famished. He said to Jacob, "Quick, let me have some of that red stew! I'm famished!" (That is why he was also called Edom.) Jacob replied, "First, sell me your birthright."
>
> "Look, I am about to die," Esau said. "What good is the birthright to me?" But Jacob said, "Swear to me first." So he swore an oath to him, selling his birthright to Jacob.
>
> Then Jacob gave Esau some bread and some lentil stew. He ate and drank and then got up and left.
>
> So Esau despised his birthright.

In Pastor Jon Courson's sermon, he says that Esau was a man who only cared about the flesh. His life was about satisfying the flesh instead of the spirit. Birthright meant not just getting double wealth, it also meant taking care of the servants and family through ministering which is feeding the spirit. This was Jacob's passion. Esau didn't care about any of it.

Jacob goes on to steal Esau's blessing as well. The story continues:

> When Esau was forty years old, he married Judith, daughter of Beeri the Hittite, and Basemath, daughter of Elon the Hittite. They were a source of grief to Isaac and Rebekah.
>
> When Isaac was old and his eyes were so weak that he could no longer see, he called for Esau his older son and said to him, "My son."

"Here I am," he answered.

Isaac said, "I am now an old man and don't know the day of my death. Now then, get your equipment—your quiver and bow—and go out to the open country to hunt some wild game for me. Prepare me the kind of tasty food I like and bring it to me to eat, so that I may give you my blessing before I die."

Now Rebekah was listening as Isaac spoke to his son Esau. When Esau left for the open country to hunt game and bring it back, Rebekah said to her son Jacob, "Look, I overheard your father say to your brother Esau, 'Bring me some game and prepare me some tasty food to eat, so that I may give you my blessing in the presence of the Lord before I die.'

"Now, my son, listen carefully and do what I tell you. Go out to the flock and bring me two choice young goats, so I can prepare some tasty food for your father, just the way he likes it. Then take it to your father to eat, so that he may give you his blessing before he dies."

Jacob's mother helped disguise her son to deceive her husband in believing he was giving his blessing to Esau. Right after Isaac had blessed Jacob, Esau returned to get his blessing. His father unbeknownst to what he had done, could not give Esau the blessing because it had been given to Jacob.

Esau held a grudge against Jacob because of the blessing his father had given him. He said to himself, "The days of mourning for my father are near; then I will kill my brother Jacob."

When Rebekah was told what her older son Esau had said, she sent for her younger son Jacob and said to him, "Your brother Esau is planning to avenge himself by killing you. Now then, my son, do what I say: Flee at once to my brother Laban in Harran. Stay with him for a while until your brother is no longer angry with you and forgets what you did to him. I'll send word for you to come back from there. Why should I lose both of you in one day?" That was the last time Rebekah saw Jacob.

Did Rebekah break the first principle in Celebrate Recovery? Did she try to be God?

She helped her son Jacob deceive his father and receive Esau's blessing. As a result, Esau threatened his brother's life which caused Jacob to go into hiding. Rebekah never saw Jacob again. What if she had needed him as our mother needed us?

What if she had needed one of her sons to become her caregiver?

The first principle in Celebrate Recovery is that we must stop acting like God. We are not God. Rebekah should not have eavesdropped on her husband when he was talking to Esau. She should not have taken matters into her own hands to make sure Jacob gets the blessing by showing him how to deceive his father. Where was her faith that if it was God's will, Jacob would receive his father's blessing?

Her actions started a feud that lasted throughout many generations, causing death, destruction, and heartaches.

It's 9:30 p.m.

I shut the physical door to my bedroom and opened my spiritual door to God.

Today, I am reading about the prophecy of Obadiah. Rebekah's actions toward one son bring turmoil for generations upon generations between two nations—the Edomites and the Israelites.

During the invasion of the Babylonians, the Israelites were taken captive. The Israelites are descendants of Jacob, whose name was changed to Israel after his encounter with God. The Edomites descendants of Esau committed a great sin in God's eyes. They didn't help their distant cousins, the Israelites, when they were being attacked. Instead, they just stood on the sidelines and then helped the Babylonians by pillaging from the Israelites. They even captured the remaining Israelites and sold them into bondage.

This led to the vision of Obadiah.

This is what the Sovereign Lord says about Edom:

> We have heard a message from the Lord: An
> envoy was sent to the nations to say, "Rise, let us
> go against her for battle.
> See, I will make you small among the nations;
> you will be utterly despised.
> The pride of your heart has deceived you,
> you who live in the clefts of the rocks
> and make your home on the heights,
> you who say to yourself,
> 'Who can bring me down to the
> ground?" Though you soar like the eagle
> and make your nest among the stars,
> from there I will bring you down,"
> declares the LORD.

I know that the LORD is referring to the Edomites when he says, "You who live in the clefts in the rocks." The Edomites dwelt in the rock city of Petra.

The Edomites had committed a great sin. They stood by and didn't help the Israelites when they were being attacked. It is said that some were actually rejoicing. In God's eyes, that was the same thing as actually committing the act against his chosen people.

It's 9:30 p.m. on Christmas Day!

Once again, I shut my bedroom door and opened my spiritual door to God!

I opened my Bible to Matthew 2:1–23. It says:

> Now when Jesus was born in Bethlehem of
> Judaea in the days of Herod the king, behold,
> there came wise men from the east to Jerusalem,

saying, "Where is he that is born King of the Jews? For we have seen his star in the east and have come to worship him."

When Herod the king had heard these things, he was troubled and all Jerusalem with him.

And when he had gathered all the chief priests and scribes of the people together, he demanded of them where Christ should be born.

And they said unto him, "In Bethlehem of Judaea: for thus it is written by the prophet, 'And thou Bethlehem, in the land of Juda, for out of thee shall come a governor that shall rule my people Israel.'"

Then Herod, when he had privily called the wise men, enquired of them diligently what time the star appeared.

And he sent them to Bethlehem, and said, "Go and search diligently for the young child; and when ye have found him, bring me word again, that I may come and worship him also."

When they had heard the king, they departed; and, lo, the star, which they saw in the east, went before them, till it came and stood over where the young child was.

When they saw the star, they rejoiced with exceeding great joy.

And when they were come into the house, they saw the young child with Mary, his mother, and fell down, and worshipped him: and when they had opened their treasures, they presented unto him gifts; gold, and frankincense, and myrrh.

And being warned of God in a dream that they should not return to Herod, they departed into their own country another way.

And when they were departed, behold, the angel of the Lord appeareth to Joseph in a dream, saying, "Arise, and take the young child and his mother, and flee into Egypt, and be thou there until I bring thee word, for Herod will seek the young child to destroy him."

When he arose, he took the young child and his mother by night, and departed into Egypt, and he was there until the death of Herod: that it might be fulfilled which was spoken of the Lord by the prophet, saying, "Out of Egypt have I called my son."

Then Herod, when he saw that he was mocked of by the wise men, was exceeding wroth, and sent forth, and slew all the children that were in Bethlehem, and in all the coasts thereof, from two years old and under, according to the time which he had diligently enquired of the wise men.

Then was fulfilled that which was spoken by Jeremy the prophet, saying, "In Rama was there a voice heard—lamentation and weeping and great mourning, Rachel weeping for her children, and would not be comforted because they are not."

But when Herod was dead, behold, an angel of the Lord appeareth in a dream to Joseph in Egypt, saying, "Arise, and take the young child and his mother, and go into the land of Israel, for they are dead which sought the young child's life."

And he arose and took the young child and his mother and came into the land of Israel.

But when he heard that Archelaus did reign in Judaea in the room of his father Herod, he was afraid to go thither: notwithstanding, being warned of God in a dream, he turned aside into the parts of Galilee.

And he came and dwelt in a city called Nazareth, that it might be fulfilled which was spoken by the prophets, He shall be called a Nazarene.

Herod had killed all children two years old and under in trying to eliminate Jesus. Herod was an Edomite.

Mother Rebekah's actions had a ripple effect all the way to the birth of Jesus! It's horrifying to try and imagine a life without Jesus who rescued us from our sins.

# CHAPTER 5

# COVID-19 Is No Match for God's Will

Heavenly Father,

I am tired of walking in darkness and wallowing in sin.

You've seen the things I've done and the places I've been.

I looked down when I should have looked up, cursed when I should have prayed, and ran when I should have kneeled.

Then, I opened the Book. I studied the Word. I will be saved I pray it is God's Will.

I fall, I get up, I stumble back into sin, then I try again.

Lord, only you know how this story ends! Amen.

It happened the day my sister called to tell me she had found a great senior community in Colorado to move into. My sister put her trailer on the market recently. She had been living there for more than twenty-five years. She was planning to live in St. Louis for six months out of the year and live in Colorado Springs for the other six months. Originally, she had planned to move to St. Louis permanently. She had decided this two years ago but never actually did it. She kept moving the date out. She had lived in Colorado for over thirty years. She recently retired from the Air Force. It was during her retirement that she said she believed God wanted her to help our mom with her nutrition. Her goal is to oversee all of Mom's meals. She said God had made this her new purpose in life since she was now retired. She must live near Mom in order to make this happen.

She decided that since she couldn't commit to making the full move, she was going to try out her plans to live in St. Louis for six months out of the year. She needed to test the waters before jumping in completely. That's what my sister had intended. That day when she called, I had a surprise for her. It was a surprise that would keep her in Colorado Springs the whole year.

I told my sister that I was coming with my mom and husband to live in Colorado Springs. I wanted to know if she had sold her trailer because I wanted to rent it.

I had been so busy focusing on what my daughter was doing that I didn't notice my mom had stopped taking her medication. Her thyroid had been removed when she was in her early twenties. She had to take medication for the rest of her life since she no longer had a thyroid. My mom started to get very sick, and I didn't know why. She had stopped eating and could barely get out of bed. I checked her pill bottle and realized she hadn't taken a pill in weeks, maybe months. It was at that very moment I knew I had failed as my mom's caregiver. I was so busy focusing on what my daughter was doing that I neglected the most important job of my life—caring for my mom.

Unfortunately, my sister said someone had put a bid on the trailer, and she accepted the offer. She said that there was a vacancy at the senior living complex where she was moving. She was very excited at the thought of us coming there to live.

I googled Affinity online to see if it was something I should consider. I never pictured us living in a senior community. It could be nice living around people close to our age. Affinity had lots of amenities. There was a library and a movie theater in the building for Mom. There was a bar and game room for my husband. And for me, it had an indoor pool and workout room. This place seemed like the answer to my prayers. It offered something for each of us. It would also be nice for Mom to socialize with people close to her age. I was eager to sign up.

I spoke to the leasing manager the following day and rented a two-bedroom and two-bathroom unit. Now how did I happen to have just the exact money in my account to put down that deposit? I don't usually have money in my account. It was all God's doing.

Unlike my sister, it didn't take me two years to pull the trigger, it only took me two months to move once God had put it on my heart.

My sister knew I was moving in less than two months. My mother knew we were moving in less than two months. And my husband knew we were moving in less than two months. The only person who didn't know was my daughter. I had to wait for the right time to tell her. I just didn't know when that time would arrive.

The following week, my daughter came home after being away for two days. She had been at the casino. She walked in the front door, and I immediately met her and told her that I was moving to Colorado Springs on April 1, 2020. She looked at me with a surprised expression. She probably thought I was coming to yell at her for being out for two days. She said okay then went into her room. I knew she had been up for two days. I couldn't tell if she was able to comprehend what I had just told her.

The next day, when my daughter came out of her bedroom, I told her again that I was moving to Colorado Springs. She asked if it was because of her staying out and not calling. I said no. I told her that she was an adult and do not have to answer to me. I explained to her that I needed my space so I can take care of my responsibilities. I told her that my mom was my number one priority, and I had let her down. I won't make that mistake again. I must leave so I can take better care of my loved ones. There was too much distraction here. I told my daughter that she needed her space as well.

Weeks had gone by after I told my daughter about my move to Colorado. The subject had not come up again. Things were happening in the news that had caught our attention. The COVID epidemic had gotten serious.

I started checking out the headlines on the coronavirus from ABC news.

## Week 1
## March 1–8

New cases confirmed that week: 487; new deaths confirmed that week: 21.

March 1: New York Gov. Andrew Cuomo announces the first COVID-19 case in the state—a woman who had traveled from Iran. Former Surgeon General Jerome Adams tweets that people should stop buying masks to prevent a shortage for health workers, adding that "They are not effective in preventing general public from catching #Coronavirus."

March 6: Ten states confirm their first cases. Adams tells Fox News the risk to the "average American remains low" and that wearing a mask "may actually increase their risk of getting coronavirus" because of people touching their faces. (Adams later clarified the position, saying they learned more about asymptomatic transmission, and the CDC in early April advised wearing non-medical masks.)

I planned to move my family across the states from St. Louis, Missouri, to Colorado Springs in three weeks! I am keeping up with the news to see if I should get face masks in order for us to go into public places to use the restroom and to buy food.

## Week 2
## March 9–15

New cases confirmed that week: 2,618; new deaths confirmed that week: 48.

March 9: The spread of the virus and its effect on businesses result in the stock market plummeting 7.79%. An automatic circuit breaker safety mechanism is activated to stop stock prices from free falling.

March 11: WHO characterizes the coronavirus outbreak as a "pandemic," marking the first pandemic caused by a coronavirus, and Trump restricts travel from Europe for thirty days. The NBA suspends its season after Utah Jazz center Rudy Gobert tested positive before tipoff.

March 12: Broadway theaters in New York City go dark. San Francisco shuts down schools. The NHL suspends its season, MLB suspends spring training, and the NCAA suspends its college basketball tournaments. The stock market saw another plunge and ended the day with a 9.99% loss. Disney (the parent company of ABC News) announces park closures.

March 13: President Trump declares a national emergency as the death toll increases, freeing up to $50 billion in funding and establishing private sector partnerships to increase testing capacity. Dr. Anthony Fauci suggests it could be "several weeks" before cases peak.

On March 15, my daughter, Eve, returned from Walmart and said, "It's a mad house out there!" People are stocking up and the shelves are getting empty. I still wasn't concerned about the move to Colorado. My plans to move in two weeks hadn't changed.

### Week 3
### March 16–22

New cases confirmed that week: 64,258; new deaths confirmed that week: 491.

March 16: New York City closes schools. The stock market begins the week with another devastating tumble and closes with a 12.93% drop. The College Board cancels May 2 SAT. President Trump urges people not to gather in groups of ten or more and avoid eating and drinking in restaurants and bars among other new guidelines, suggesting that this "sacrifice" will help avoid putting the vulnerable in "harm's way."

March 17: All fifty states report at least one coronavirus case. New York City and Los Angeles shut down movie theaters, and Pfizer and BioNTech announce they will team up to develop a vaccine. Six counties in Northern California ordered to "shelter in place."

March 18: Macy's and other major retailers temporarily close their stores.

March 19: California Gov. Gavin Newsom becomes the first governor in the country to release a stay-at-home order for non-essential workers, saying the move was "necessary" and "open-ended."

March 20: Cuomo issues his "New York State on Pause" order, closing all non-essential businesses. The order was effective March 22.

My daughter hadn't been to the casino in over a week. She commented that I had no reason to move now that the casinos have shut their doors. I tried to get her to understand that there was more to my moving than just her addiction. I explained to her that everything's not always about her. I had to move to Colorado for many reasons, I believed mainly for me and my mother's health. We had been living on fast food and junk food. Our nutrition was extremely poor. I always felt sickly. How on earth could I be an effective caregiver when I needed to be cared for? I hoped that it would be easier to break bad habits if I got out of the environment that had caused them.

## Week 4
## March 23–31

New cases confirmed that week: 146,165; new deaths confirmed that week: 4,555.

March 24: Army hospital units are deployed to New York state to deal with declining hospital capacity. Army engineers start converting the Javits Center into a temporary field hospital able to house nearly 3,000 beds, making it one of the largest in the US.

March 25: Congress strikes a deal and approves a $2 trillion stimulus deal that gives most adult Americans a $1,200 check. Trump suggests "large sections" of the country could get back to "normal" sooner than others.

During the fourth week of March, my daughter and I watched episodes of *The Walking Dead*. We were on lockdown. We thought it was a good time to catch up on some of our favorite television shows.

March 26: The US surpasses China with the most confirmed coronavirus cases in the world, topping 82,000 cases.

March 27: The US surpasses 100,000 total cases.

My daughter and I watched the latest episodes of *Grey's Anatomy* once we finished watching *The Walking Dead*. We watched the episode where Richard's wife was diagnosed with Alzheimer's. We could sympathize with what Richard was going through. We understood the hard decisions he had to make regarding the wellbeing of both him and his wife. He was fortunate to have known someone who had gone through what he was going through. He was able to get valuable advice and guidance from a friend. It made all the difference for both the caregiver and the one receiving the care. His wife would leave food cooking on the stove and wander off. She needed to be watched 24/7. It was a big step for Richard to realize it was not safe for him or his wife to keep her at home. He placed her in a care facility that was recommended by his friend.

March 30: US Navy ship arrives in New York City to help relieve pressure on local hospitals.

March 31: Twenty-six states and territories have issued stay-at-home orders.

I needed to make things right with my daughter. I couldn't leave with things being the way they were. There was so much tension between us. I always wanted to have a close relationship with my one and only child. Today, I would settle for at least a cordial one. During the stay-at-home order, we worked together, cooking, cleaning, and taking care of my mom and husband. We talked and watched television. We read the Bible and watched church on YouTube. I had never spent this much time with my daughter since she was born.

It's April 1. I was supposed to be moving into the Affinity Senior Living apartment complex today. Instead, my mom, husband, and I are still in Missouri due to the stay-at-home order, though I never once considered it a sign that I shouldn't move. In the meantime, I was making amends with my daughter. I didn't want to leave with her so mad at me that we stopped talking. We had spent thirty days together. It was therapy for both of us. As I kept up with the latest headlines in the news, I made my decision to move by May 1 no matter what. My daughter told me that she could not help me move to Colorado because it would be too hard on her. She said she couldn't believe I would move my eighty-year-old mom during a pandemic. I replied that our bodies are immune because this is God's will. My daughter then said, "What if this is happening as a sign that you shouldn't move?" I replied, "Satan is always working to sabotage God's will."

I just knew in my heart I had to do this whether my daughter accepted it or not. It was going to happen.

*8:18 p.m. ET, April 4, 2020*

On Saturday, at least 27,867 new cases were reported and at least 1,139 new deaths in the US have been reported, according to a tally by Johns Hopkins.

*8:45 p.m. ET, April 4, 2020*

"This is very important—the next two weeks are extraordinarily important, and that's why I think you've heard from Dr. (Anthony) Fauci, from myself, from the president, and the vice president that this is the moment to do everything that you can on the presidential guidelines," Birx said. "This is the moment to not be going to the grocery store, not going to the pharmacy, but doing everything you can to keep your family and your friends safe, and that means everybody doing the six-feet distancing, washing your hands." Birx made her comments at the daily coronavirus task briefing at the White House.

*8:46 p.m. ET, April 4, 2020*

"US marks record for most new coronavirus deaths reported in a single day," reports CNN's Hollie Silverman

It's April 15. Rent is due at Affinity. I called the manager to explain I couldn't move there on April 1 due to the stay-at-home order. The manager waived April's rent. Meanwhile, my daughter and I were getting along better than we had previously. Headlines on the epidemic started to look promising. I could see a pathway opening for my family and me. I knew I would be moving at the end of April. I began to finish packing.

*3:00 p.m. April 20, 2020*

Pennsylvania will begin reopening the economy on May 8. Pennsylvania governor Tom Wolf on Monday said the state is going to move towards reopening its economy on May 8. Wolf announced small steps like allowing curbside liquor sales and starting construction projects while maintaining social distancing guidelines.

"We cannot relax," he says. "We're going to continue to take precautions that limit our physical contact with others, cutting down transmission links while we move toward an opening on May 8."

*Updated 5:38 p.m. / April 20, 2020*

Gyms, bowling alleys, and salons will reopen in Georgia on Friday, a report by Victoria Albert says. Georgia governor Brian Kemp announced Monday that a number of non-essential businesses including gyms, bowling alleys, and salons will be allowed to reopen this Friday, according to CBS affiliate WTOC.

Kemp also said he plans to allow restaurants to reopen dine-in services by next Monday as long as they meet specific guidelines that will be announced later in the week.

"The entities which I am reopening are not reopening as business as usual," Kemp said. "Each of these entities will be subject to specific restrictions including adherence to the minimal basic operations, social distancing, and regular sanitation."

Eve and I watched episodes of *The Blacklist*. The relationship between the father and daughter resembled the relationship between Eve and me. I could identify with Red. He wanted to protect his daughter by staying away from her. I am detrimental to Eve by being around her. I can't say no to the things I should say no to. I always want to please her no matter what the cost may be. I do this because I feel that I had neglected her when she was growing up. I was so busy going to college to pursue a career that I missed some important events in my daughter's life. Now that she's an adult, I want to make up for those lost years. I believed that my moving away is the best thing I can do for my daughter as well as for myself and my mother.

I started packing for the move two weeks ago. My daughter, Eve, still insisted that she would not help me with the move. I called my grandson to tell him when I needed to rent the U-Haul truck. He told me to talk to his mom about it. I didn't need to talk to his mom because God had this.

I would be ready to leave St. Louis on April 29.

April 22: Expert says it's not too soon to make plans to restart the economy, but life won't be the same when we do (Boston Globe).

To reopen the economy during the COVID-19 pandemic, planning could address known risks, such as people being in close proximity and in large groups and building characteristics such as room layouts that allow the separation of people, said Harvey Fineberg, president of the Gordon and Betty Moore Foundation and former dean of Harvard Chan School, at a recent forum organized by the school and the New England Journal of Medicine. He predicted that, as the economy gets rolling, handshakes will be a waning custom, and people will wear face masks. "In my opinion, life in the time of coronavirus is not never going to be quite the same as life prior to the coronavirus," he said. Another panelist, Caroline Buckee, associate professor of epidemiology, said that more testing—both diagnostic tests to see who's infected and antibody testing to determine the extent of the epidemic—is crucial to reopening. "I wouldn't be considering opening up society until I had testing in place. Period," she said.

The morning of April 29, my grandsons packed up the U-Haul, my daughter packed up the SUV, and we headed toward Colorado. I couldn't believe how empty the highways were. When we stopped to get something to eat, the lines were extremely long because no one was allowed to go inside. We put on our masks when we went into the gas stations to use the restrooms. There were some stations that had run out of gas. I felt like we were headed into an apocalypse.

The outside world looked much different. The few who were out had their faces covered. There was an unpleasant silence. People seemed lonely and afraid. They kept their distance.

April 30: Expert report predicts up to two more years of pandemic misery, CNN reports.

A team of pandemic experts has predicted in a new report that the new coronavirus is likely to keep spreading for another eighteen to twenty-four months in the US. They urged officials to stop telling people that the pandemic is on the wane and instead to prepare for a long period of intense effort to quell upcoming waves of disease. Epidemiologist Marc Lipsitch, coauthor of the report, expressed surprise that many states are lifting restrictions aimed at curbing the spread of COVID-19. "I think it's an experiment that likely will cost lives, especially in places that do it without careful controls to try to figure out when to try to slow things down again," he said.

April 30: It doesn't stay where you started: Reopening some states heightens the risk of coronavirus surges in others, STAT reports.

As some states begin to reopen their economies, and more people move around and come into contact with others, coronavirus infections may resurge. And if people travel, the infection could spread to other states. These potential ripple effects could also occur if universities, employers, or sports leagues decide to reopen. If universities bring students back—reasoning that, overall, they're less impacted by COVID-19—"and young people start transmitting among themselves but largely asymptomatically or with mild symptoms, if you don't look deep enough at the question, you might say, 'Great, we're building up herd immunity,'" said epidemiologist Michael Mina. "But then those young people will inevitably start seeding outbreaks to the wider community, and anyone else can be at risk."

On April 30, 2020, my daughter had moved my mom, husband, and me safely from St. Louis, Missouri, to Colorado Springs. It took two grandsons, two days, one U-Haul, and an SUV. I never doubted it would happen any other way than by the grace of God!

# CHAPTER 6

# Life at Affinity

It's Mother's Day.

We have been living at Affinity for ten days.

My sister and I bought Mom's favorite flowers to decorate her new home. Mom believes she is spending Mother's Day on vacation at a resort. My sister and I surrounded her with beautiful flower arrangements to take pictures with and send to her grandchildren. We couldn't take Mom out to dinner because restaurants were not at full service yet in Colorado. Social gatherings are limited to ten to twenty-five. The latest update reports that a hundred thousand Americans have died from coronavirus complications. Colorado reported 1421 deaths out of 25,121 COVID-19 cases. Some restaurants were offering takeout meals to help families celebrate Mother's Day.

Mom wanted barbecue ribs. My sister ordered takeout. She made homemade ice cream for dessert.

My mom is now being cared for by both of her daughters. We wanted to help our Mom. We were discussing plans for her meals. She is going from fast food in St. Louis to home-cooked meals in Colorado.

My sister, who has studied health and wellness most of her adult life, will be strict on Mom's diet after Mother's Day. She believes that if it's possible, she will be able to reverse Mom's dementia with good nutrition and Shaklee vitamins. Mom will be taken off fast food and processed foods. I am very happy about that. I have a hard time saying no to Mom when it comes to junk food. I am the daughter that gives in to Mom's wants to make her life as pleasurable as possible. My sister's main goal is to treat Mom's health issues with what she needs and not what she wants. I admire what my sister is doing for our mom. Though I still struggle with the importance of Mom's happiness, which can sometimes be detrimental to her health like Sprite sodas. She likes her McDonald's fish sandwiches and Sprite soda. She enjoys her donuts and coffee. She loves ice cream. My sister will be the bad cop. I will be the good cop. I know, if you really look at it the correct way, I am really the bad cop. I really want my sister to replace Mom's comfort food with healthy choices. I know the best way she is going to make this happen is by keeping the junk food out of the house. Everyone will eat healthy including my husband. We need this! We need it badly!

Life in Colorado Springs starts at 7:00 a.m. I start with a prayer followed by a scripture reading. By 8:00 a.m., I give Mom her prescription medication and her Shaklee supplements, which include alfalfa, vitamin D, and a multivitamin. She then must wait one hour before she can eat. I make breakfast for my husband and Mom at 9:00 a.m. Mom eats at the dining room table while watching her favorite television show *The Golden Girls*. By 10:00 a.m., she is still sitting at the dining room table where she enjoys reading her Reader's Digest or creating phrases out of the letters to her scrabble board game. After lunch, sometimes Mom and I take a walk through the lobby or outside depending on the weather and how she is feeling.

Life at Affinity is very nice, although many of the public areas such as the bar, movie theater, and game rooms have been shut down due to the coronavirus. I enjoy sitting in the beautifully-decorated lobby. I enjoy looking out the windows at the snow-peak mountains. The neighbors always speak as they walk by. Everyone here seems very friendly, although they never get too close. I can never see their smiles because of the face masks, but the tone in their voice tells me they are smiling.

My sister lives in the same building but two levels up and on the opposite side of the building. She comes down around 3:00 p.m. to take Mom to the store with her. We like to get Mom outside at least twice a week. Mom always wonders why we are still on vacation. Every time my sister takes Mom out and brings her back, Mom never wants to get out of the car. She can't seem to understand that this is her new home.

My sister starts dinner at 6:00 p.m. After dinner, Mom and I find an action movie or comedy to watch before bed. Sometimes, my sister stays to watch a movie with us.

Saturdays are a little different. I don't cook on Saturdays because of Sabbath. We have a bowl of fresh fruit for breakfast, a sandwich and/or salad for lunch, and Friday's leftovers for dinner. It is also my sister's day off. Mom and I watch church on TV until 2:00 p.m. We then would sit at the dining room table and talk about any and everything. I liked to listen to my mom talk about when she was younger. I notice that her stories are getting crossed. She thinks her mother had ten girls and 2 boys. When I asked my mom what the names of her brothers are, she gives me the names of her two sons. My mother confused her sons with being my grandmother's sons. My grandmother had ten girls and no boys.

My mom and I had something very special in common. We both loved to write poems and songs. I wanted us to write a song together. We knew how much my grandmother loved the song "Amazing Grace." I told Mom we should create a version with Grandma in mind. We came up with these lyrics:

> Heavenly Father,
> My grandmother was my "Amazing Grace."
> When things became unbearable, she would
> lead me to you!
> She raised me in a home full of warm embrace
> that kept me going, kept me pulling through!
>
> Heavenly Father,
> My mother has been my "Amazing Grace."
> When I wallowed in pity, she didn't come
> to console

> She brought a poem that put a smile on
> my face
> letting me know that God is in control!
>
> Heavenly Father,
> My life is filled with "Amazing Grace."
> I cry then laugh. I fall then rise. I kick and
> fuss then pray
> God answered my prayers in amazing ways
> Sending blessings to me day after day.

I wanted to do an activity with Mom at least twice a week. I enjoyed working on poems or creating a family album with her. We would sit at the dining room table for hours.

Life at Affinity showed me that I could take care of my loved ones on my own. I had to sacrifice my travel business. My mom was my priority.

My sister and I would always find time to discuss Mom's wellbeing. We both wanted what was best for her. We both had our assignments. I took on the job of keeping Mom entertained while my sister worked on her nutrition. I wanted happiness for my mom, and my sister wanted longevity for our mom. She and I wanted our mom to have both of course. I was just better at pleasing her while my sister was better at healing her.

My sister is putting everyone on a twenty-one-day sugar detox. I don't eat many sweets, but my sister and mother have a major sweet tooth. As a result, sugar is being removed from our meals completely for the next twenty-one days. My sister printed out the menu for the first week which looked pretty good.

My sister gave me a copy of the Sugar Detox Food Menu for the first week. Breakfast will either consist of bacon and eggs or a smoothie. My sister doesn't like for Mom to eat bacon, but if she's giving up sugar, I needed to at least keep her favorite breakfast during this detox. Bacon is on the *Yes* list of foods she can have. My sister took out all the sugar in the apartment. There will be no sugar to make Mom coffee. I know she will ask for it every morning. Every morning I will say we don't have any sugar.

Lunch for day one consisted of grilled chicken and a fresh garden salad with pecans. Dinner consisted of grilled salmon and asparagus. Day two lunch was mushroom soup and mixed greens salad. Dinner for day two consisted of ginger-garlic chicken thighs, cauliflower rice, and broccoli. Day three lunch consisted of a spinach salad and two boiled eggs. Dinner for day three was baked cod, cauliflower rice, and asparagus. Day four lunch was Portabella burgers and mixed green salad. Dinner was hot wings, cucumber salad, and zoodles. Day five lunch was chicken tortilla soup. Dinner was shepherd's pie and fried cabbage. Day six lunch was veggie stir fry over cauliflower rice and Asian greens. Dinner for day six was T-bone steak, steamed broccoli, and mixed greens salad. Day seven lunch was tomato soup and spinach salad. Dinner was leftovers from day four dinner.

It took a lot of hard work and time for my sister to plan the food menu. I knew the planning would be the most important process for this to work. I gave kudos to my sister.

Day 0—here we go! Mom didn't have any idea what we were getting ready to do. I did and started to feel anxiety, fear, and excitement as my sister and I prepared for the twenty-one-day detox.

Day 1—ready and willing! I didn't experience anything different on day one but still positive. Mom was still talking about signing herself into a nursing home as she walked from her bedroom to the living room, which was about eleven steps.

Day 2—no difference! It just seems like a normal day. Being prepared was the key to getting off on the right foot.

Day 3—Mom's withdrawal. She seems a bit fatigued. I think she has caught a bug. My sister says Mom will get better. She is just experiencing sugar withdrawal.

Day 4—three days down, eighteen to go! This new eating schedule has affected Mom's mood more than I had anticipated. She is very irritable. I try to find some magazines with positive articles for her to read. I keep them on the dining table where she likes to sit and stare out of the glass door to the balcony.

Day 5—she still doesn't seem to be getting the hang of this. Mom keeps asking for Honey Nut Cheerios. I am so glad we cleared all the processed foods out of the apartment. There is nothing for her to find in the kitchen that will break her detox. I know she can do this.

Day 6—Mom wants to go to McDonald's to get two fish sandwiches and a large Sprite. Her bad habits are still lingering. I asked my sister to buy more green-tip bananas since Mom seems to like them.

Day 7—almost a whole week down! Both Mom and I have little constipation going on. My sister gave us some Shaklee Herb Lax that helped.

Day 8—two more weeks to go! Mom still seems a little fatigue. We are still on track, without any slipups so far.

Day 9—I'm getting bored eating the same thing. I must give it to Mom; she doesn't complain about eating the same thing because she never remembers what she had the day before. However, I am tired of the same foods. I need my sister to get creative with meal planning.

Day 10—almost at the halfway point. My sister is going to make some lettuce wraps tonight. That will be something different. I am excited to try it. I am really excited about dinner! Now, I need to try and get Mom as excited. By the way, she hasn't asked for McDonald's in two days.

Day 11—Mom and I are doing this! The lettuce wraps were very good last night. Mom walked to the mailbox with me today and didn't have to stop halfway like she usually does. She was excited to get her Reader's Digest to read. I noticed that Mom has been smiling more than frowning the past couple of days. This makes me happy!

Day 12—smooth sailing! Mom hasn't asked if we have any ice cream. Her sugar craving seems to have waned. She hasn't signed herself in a nursing home yet! Could we be on to a new way of eating forever?

Day 13—there are some changes happening! Mom said she slept like a baby last night! She is walking slightly more upright and with fewer moans and groans.

Day 14—only one week left! I have taken good notes through-out this experience. I will be able to refer to them when I want to get motivated for round two.

Day 15—it's good to not do it alone! My sister has been looking at other resources and trying new recipes to make this easy for Mom and me. I don't think Mom and I could have lasted through this without her.

Day 16—reaping the benefits! I weighed this morning and have lost eight pounds. I can see my shoes. LOL. Mom is rolling up her pants because they are too big. We didn't do the detox to lose weight, although it's one of the great benefits.

Day 17—the finish line is within sight! I am already trying to plan what foods I will add once this detox is over. I don't plan to go back to my old habits of cookies and ice cream several times a week. I realize it's easier said than done.

Day 18—trying not to ruin a good thing! I have started think-ing about what I want to eat on Day twenty-two. I know what I want to drink—a raspberry mocha from Dutch Brothers. The caffeine is calling!

Day 19—three more days and counting! Mom and I will finish strong. I couldn't believe my ears. Mom is talking about getting a part-time job. What a drastic change in mindset!

Day 2—only one day left! Mom and I are still doing good. Mom never really knew she was doing a sugar detox. She was just eating what her daughters prepared for her. She's a real trooper.

Day 21—we made it! It's always a good feeling when you com-plete anything in life. I know my body thanks me for it. I don't know if this detox did anything to help with Mom's dementia. She never stopped seeing images outside that weren't there.

Day 22—nothing too crazy! Mom had the usual breakfast. The only thing different is that I gave her coffee with her bacon and eggs. I did it because she asked for it. Every time she sees someone on tele-vision drinking coffee, she wants a cup. Remember, I am the daugh-ter that gives in to Mom's wants. I am still a work in progress!

Day 23—I liked the way I felt physically after the twenty-one-day sugar detox. I realized how important it was to keep a positive frame of mind when caring for someone with Alzheimer's. I liked how I was able to handle my mom's outburst with patience instead of frustration. I am still trying to learn as much as I can about Mom's condition. I haven't been able to identify what stage of dementia she's currently at. Earlier, I identified the three stages taken from the Alzheimer's Association website. Here it's a little more broken down into five instead of three stages. I really believe she's in the fourth stage. The following information was taken from the Mayo Clinic Staff online posting on the five stages of Alzheimer's:

There are five stages associated with Alzheimer's disease: preclinical Alzheimer's disease, mild cognitive impairment due to Alzheimer's disease, mild dementia due to Alzheimer's disease, moderate dementia due to Alzheimer's disease, and severe dementia due to Alzheimer's disease. Dementia is a term used to describe a group of symptoms that affect intellectual and social abilities severely enough to interfere with daily function.

The five Alzheimer's stages can help you understand what might happen, but it's important to know that these stages are only rough generalizations. The disease is a continuous process. Each person has a different experience with Alzheimer's and its symptoms.

*Stage One: Preclinical Alzheimer's Disease:*

Alzheimer's disease begins long before any symptoms become apparent. This stage is called preclinical Alzheimer's disease, and it's usually identified only in research settings. You won't notice symptoms during this stage nor will those around you.

This stage of Alzheimer's can last for years, possibly even decades. Although you won't notice any changes, new imaging technologies can now identify deposits of a protein called amyloid-beta that is a hallmark of Alzheimer's disease. The ability to identify these early deposits may be especially important for clinical trials and in the future as new treatments are developed for Alzheimer's disease.

*Stage Two: Mild Cognitive Impairment (MCI) due to Alzheimer's Disease:*

People with mild cognitive impairment have mild changes in their memory and thinking ability. These changes aren't significant enough to affect work or relationships yet. People with MCI may have memory lapses when it comes to information that is usually easily remembered such as conversations, recent events, or appointments.

People with MCI may also have trouble judging the amount of time needed for a task, or they may have difficulty correctly judging the number or sequence of steps needed to complete a task. The ability to make sound decisions can become harder for people with MCI.

Not everyone with mild cognitive impairment has Alzheimer's disease. MCI is often diagnosed based on the doctor's review of symptoms and professional judgment. But, if necessary, the same procedures used to identify pre-clinical Alzheimer's disease can help determine whether MCI is due to Alzheimer's disease or something else.

*Stage Three: Mild Dementia Due to Alzheimer's Disease*

Alzheimer's disease is often diagnosed in the mild dementia stage, when it becomes clear to family and doctors that a person is having significant trouble with memory and thinking that impacts daily functioning.

In the mild dementia stage, people may experience:

- Memory loss of recent events. Individuals may have an especially hard time remembering newly learned information and ask the same question over and over.
- Difficulty with problem-solving, complex tasks, and sound judgments. Planning a family event or balancing a checkbook may become overwhelming. Many people experience lapses in judgment such as when making financial decisions.
- Changes in personality. People may become subdued or withdrawn—especially in socially challenging situations—or show uncharacteristic irritability or anger. Reduced motivation to complete tasks also is common.
- Difficulty organizing and expressing thoughts. Finding the right words to describe objects or clearly express ideas becomes increasingly challenging.
- Getting lost or misplacing belongings. Individuals have increasing trouble finding their way around even in familiar places. It's also common to lose or misplace things including valuable items.

*Stage Four: Moderate Dementia Due to Alzheimer's Disease*

During the moderate dementia stage of Alzheimer's disease, people grow more confused and forgetful and begin to need more help with daily activities and self-care.

People with the moderate dementia stage of Alzheimer's disease may:

- Show increasingly poor judgment and deepening confusion. Individuals lose track of where they are, the day of the week or the season. They may confuse family members or close friends with one another or mistake strangers for family.
- Wander, possibly in search of surroundings that feel more familiar. These difficulties make it unsafe to leave those in the moderate dementia stage on their own.
- Experience even greater memory loss. People may forget details of their personal history, such as their address or phone number, or where they attended school. They repeat favorite stories or make up stories to fill gaps in memory.
- Need help with some daily activities. Assistance may be required with choosing proper clothing for the occasion or the weather and with bathing, grooming, using the bathroom, and other self-care. Some individuals occasionally lose control of their bladder or bowel movements.
- Undergo significant changes in personality and behavior. It's not unusual during the moderate dementia stage for people to

develop unfounded suspicions—for example, to become convinced that friends, family, or professional caregivers are stealing from them or that a spouse is having an affair. Others may see or hear things that aren't really there.

- Grow restless or agitated, especially late in the day. Some people may have outbursts of aggressive physical behavior.

*Stage Five: Severe Dementia Due to Alzheimer's Disease*

In the late stage of the disease, which is called severe dementia due to Alzheimer's disease, mental function continues to decline, and the disease has a growing impact on movement and physical capabilities.

In late-stage severe dementia due to Alzheimer's disease, people generally:

- Lose the ability to communicate coherently. An individual can no longer converse or speak in ways that make sense, although he or she may occasionally say words or phrases.
- Require daily assistance with personal care. This includes total assistance with eating, dressing, using the bathroom, and all other daily self-care tasks.
- Experience a decline in physical abilities. A person may become unable to walk without assistance, then unable to sit or hold up his or her head without support. Muscles may become rigid and reflexes abnormal. Eventually, a person loses the ability to swallow and to control bladder and bowel functions.

*Rate of Progression through Alzheimer's Disease Stages:*

The rate of progression for Alzheimer's disease varies widely. On average, people with Alzheimer's disease live between three and eleven years after diagnosis, but some survive twenty years or more. The degree of impairment at diagnosis can affect life expectancy. Untreated vascular risk factors such as hypertension are associated with a faster rate of progression of Alzheimer's disease.

Pneumonia is a common cause of death because impaired swallowing allows food or beverages to enter the lungs, where an infection can begin. Other common causes of death include dehydration, malnutrition, falls, and other infections.

# CHAPTER 7

# The Shades Go Down Quickly on FalconView

Our lease at Affinity ended in March 2021. My sister and I decided that life would be much easier if she lived in the same apartment with us. We found a great three-bedroom, three-bath apartment. It was a perfect place with plenty of space. My sister had a private bedroom, bath, and walk-in closet upstairs. Mom's bedroom was on the first floor across from the main bathroom. My and my husband's bedroom was also downstairs not far from Mom's. What attracted my sister and me to the apartment was the panoramic view of the mountains outside our kitchen and living room windows. It made me feel like I was in Colorado. There were plenty of windows throughout the apartment with majestic views of the Rockies.

This apartment really had Mom believing she was on vacation at another resort. She kept saying it was a beautiful place and asking how long we were staying. We couldn't get her to understand that we lived here. Mom would pack up the covers off her bed every morning. She would also pack her clothes that were in the closet. I had to remove most of her clothes and all her luggage. I left her with only three outfits to pack every day.

I was excited to have such a large bedroom, which I also turned into an office. I started working on my travel business. I loved planning trips for people. It had gotten slow during COVID-19.

However, people started making reservations in the spring of 2021 to visit America's national parks. They were tired of being locked up in the house the previous year. Everyone was ready to get out and explore. I was more than ready to send them.

I missed planning vacations for people. It brought me much enjoyment. I remember how I felt when I planned cruises for my family and me. The planning was just as enjoyable as taking the actual trip. I always considered anticipation a major part of the trip.

I was also happy to get back to work to meet people. I know only my sister in Colorado. I had become lonely, especially now. My husband fell a few weeks ago and broke his hip. He was now in a nursing facility for rehabilitation.

My sister had been in Colorado for over thirty years. She had a lot of friends to visit. I had no one. It will be nice to listen to my guests share with me what's on their bucket list so I can help make their dreams come true. The secondary benefit would be to make a friend or two.

Once I started to work again, I realized how much I missed the excitement of going on a vacation. I immediately planned a three-day getaway for my mom, sister, and me. We were taking the train from Denver to Glenwood Springs for a couple of days. I invited my daughter and her boyfriend to go with us.

I was also hoping that by taking Mom on vacation, she will see FalconView as home when we returned. I knew it was a long shot, but it was worth a shot.

It started bringing back good memories as I booked the family's vacation to Glenwood Springs. I wanted it to be perfect. I booked a one-bedroom suite. I figured if Mom wasn't up to going sightseeing, she would at least have a beautiful hotel room to relax in and order room service.

I chose Glenwood Springs for our vacation because it was only a few hours away on the train from Denver. We would enjoy a nice short train ride through the mountains to a small town nestled in the Rockies.

Wednesday, June 30, 2021, arrived.

The time was 6:00 a.m.

The phone rang. It was the front desk giving us a wake-up call.

Mom was the first to go into the bathroom to get washed and dressed.

We all were excited because most of us had never ridden on a train before.

We spent the night at Holiday Inn Express in Denver. We wanted to be close to the train station on the day we departed for Glenwood Springs.

I was so happy that my mom was getting around well. I wanted to bring the wheelchair for her, but it would not fit in the car. She only had her walking cane. She did very well walking into the hotel last night. I gave my sister credit for my mom's new diet and Shaklee supplements. Mom had been walking more upright than when she lived in St. Louis. I honestly believed that the twenty-one-day sugar detox improved Mom's physical health tremendously. Mom stopped talking about signing herself into a nursing home.

Mom's everyday conversations changed from her talking about how she inherited her mom's rheumatism to her thinking about getting a part-time job. It was truly a blessing how far she had come since we moved to Colorado from St. Louis. The only negative out of this was that she kept trying to take a cab home. We couldn't get Mom to understand that she now lived in Colorado. My mom had lived in East St. Louis and St. Louis for eighty years. Why on earth did I ever think she could see Colorado as her home?

The Denver train station was big. Mom and I hadn't walked this much in years. It wasn't bad on us though. Could it have been that we were so excited about our train ride that we didn't notice how we were feeling? I enjoyed watching Mom sip on her coffee as she studied the people who came in and went out of the Denver train station. She was amazed at how much luggage people took with them on vacation.

Mom had no idea of where we were taking her; she was just happy to be going somewhere with her daughters and granddaughter. The look of excitement in her eyes was priceless to me. I wished I could afford to take her on a vacation every other month.

The train arrived at the Denver station about twenty minutes late. We went outside to board the train. My mom and I were the last to board. We sat together on the lower level. She seemed very excited as she stared out the window when the train started to move. Mom became amazed as she looked out the window at the many trees on the mountain slopes. She said, "Look at all those people climbing the mountain. I wonder what keeps them from falling back down." I would tell her that they weren't people; those were trees. She would take another look and agree that those were trees and not people. Twenty minutes later, she would say, "Look at all those people climbing the mountain. I wonder what keeps them from falling back down." I didn't correct her after she said it the third time. I just wondered how on earth my mom could mistake trees for people. I wondered if her sight was declining rapidly. I was glad my sister had made an appointment for Mom to see the eye doctor when we return home from vacation.

The train crawled along. It crept around and through the mountains again and again. It reminded me of an old lady with a walking cane, moving slow and steady.

Mom never complained as she sat on the train for hours. My sister and my daughter sat on the upper level. They brought us lunch from the food cart. I handed Mom headphones that were playing her favorite songs. Mom was eating and humming as she enjoyed the mac and cheese.

The train conductor got on the intercom and challenged the travelers with a math problem. He said, "If the train left Chicago at 5:00 a.m. on Tuesday, traveling at thirty-five miles per hour and making a thirty-minute stop in Denver and a fifteen-minute stop in Glenwood Springs, when would that train arrive in Emeryville?" He said something like that, maybe not exactly word-for-word. I wasn't interested, so I didn't listen too carefully.

My sister, however, loved a challenge. She recently retired from the Air Force a couple of years ago as a lieutenant colonel. It's probably been a while since anyone had challenged her. She was one of the passengers who solved the problem and received a prize.

I enjoyed listening to the conductor giving us a little history of the town we were headed to. He even talked about the historic hotel in Glenwood Springs and the president who used to stay there. Resource says:

> Hotel Colorado is a historic hotel built in 1893 by Walter Devereux—a silver baron and one of the early settlers of Glenwood Springs. People came to the town on a promise of a fortune built on gold and silver mining. There were also those who came to get away from bustling city life.
>
> Glenwood Springs, notable for its healing hot springs, was brimming with potential as a destination for travelers and locals alike—and early settlers capitalized on this potential. Devereux sought to attract the wealthy and elite to his "Grande Dame," as Hotel Colorado was fondly called at the time. A 185-foot-tall fountain of water marked the center of the courtyard, and a European-style spa was an attractive draw for health-seekers during the early years of Hotel Colorado. No expense was spared in the construction of the hotel, which included amenities and attractions like tennis courts, a Victorian garden, a bird sanctuary, and a stunning indoor waterfall. The hotel has been used as a temporary White House, as a place of healing for the US Navy during the World War II years, and a community focal point from its inception. Ownership changed hands frequently until the early 1990s, when the hotel was gradually built. Despite the fact that Glenwood Springs is nearly a thousand miles from the nearest ocean, the hotel was leased to the United States Navy for use as a hospital. Named the US Naval Convalescent

Hospital, it was commissioned on July 5, 1943, and served patients until the end of the war. By the time it was decommissioned in 1946, over 6,500 patients had passed through its doors.

According to Bill Kight, executive director of the Glenwood Springs Historical Society, the hotel wasn't just a hospital. A quirk in naval law requires that any location where sailors are stationed also requires a naval prison known as a brig, and the Hotel Colorado was no exception. A room in the basement held eight prisoner cells, only five by seven feet. All evidence restored to its former glory. Most of the brig is now gone, but some Glenwood Springs residents claim that the bars were in place as late as 1974.

*President Theodore "Teddy" Roosevelt*

In 1905, Hotel Colorado became the temporary home for the president of the United States and his assistants during a three-week bear hunting expedition. Already a fan of the state of Colorado, Roosevelt stayed at the Hotel Colorado on multiple occasions.

On a three-week trip in January 1901, the then vice president hunted mountain lion on the Keystone Ranch near Meeker. It was reported by his guide that Colonel Roosevelt hung over a cliff to shoot a wounded lion between the eyes. Roosevelt's first trip to Glenwood Springs delighted him so much that he returned year after year.

According to legend, the world's most irresistible toy, the teddy bear, received its birth at Hotel Colorado. To cheer Theodore Roosevelt after an unsuccessful day of hunting, Hotel

Colorado maids presented him with a stuffed bear pieced together with scraps of fine material. Later, when he did bag a bear, his daughter Alyce admired it and said, "I will call it Teddy." The term caught on and became the name for the world's most popular toy—the Teddy bear. You can purchase one today at Hotel Colorado. It would make a nice collectible to remember your visit.

We arrived at Glenwood Springs about six hours later. We had reservations at Hotel Denver, which was just across the street from the train station. My mom, sister, and I stayed in a gorgeous one-bedroom suite. It had high-beamed ceilings and hardwood floors. There was a sofa and two wingback chairs in the living room. Mom and I slept in the bedroom, and my sister slept on the sofa in the living room.

The following day, we walked around the small town. My mom did some shopping. We stopped and had lunch outside. We didn't do much sightseeing in Glenwood Springs. We just enjoyed each other's company. It was the perfect little getaway. The second night, my mom, sister, and I sat outside the hotel and had ice cream. We watched the people walk by. Mom and I tried to distinguish the tourist from the locals. We had so much fun doing nothing.

I couldn't believe what I saw and heard when we took the train back to Denver. I needed to pinch myself. Was I dreaming! Mom was sitting next to me on the train. She took out a pen and piece of paper. She was planning how to start saving for her next vacation. Mom looked over at me and said, "I really enjoyed my vacation. Thank you for a wonderful vacation!" It was a priceless moment I will always cherish! I want to give my mom a life full of adventure for as long as she's able to enjoy it. Her happiness means the world to me. My sister and I made a good team. She worked with Mom's health so that Mom could enjoy the adventure I took her on.

Back at FalconView, I was excited to tell my new friend all about my vacation with my mother. I met him a few weeks ago on

Facebook. We discovered that we had so much in common. His wife, like my mother, also had Alzheimer's. He had given me so much good advice about how to communicate with my mom. He was the one who told me I shouldn't correct my mom about things that aren't life-threatening, like her packing up her room and asking me to call her a cab. He suggested that I respond by saying okay and walk away because she will forget. He said that correcting her all the time will only frustrate both of us.

I couldn't wait to get back to tell him how my trip to Glenwood Springs went. It's so nice to have someone to talk to who understands my situation.

The following dialogue is a sample of our communication on Messenger:

> Me: Boot camp was a nightmare, but I am so glad I did it.
> Friend: Made you stronger.
> Me: Absolutely…and disciplined. Did you serve in the military?
> Friend: No. I wish I had. I had other things going on.
> Me: Like what?
> Friend: I was involved in church and raising my kids and their mother.
> Me: Okay. You were a family man. I love it.
> Friend: Yes, I was.
> Me: That's beautiful. Are you proud of your children? Are you happy with what they have become as adults?
> Friend: Yes, I am.
> Me: Awesome.
> Friend: My daughter and her husband own a pawnshop. My son works in television.
> Me: Oh, wow! As long as they are happy doing what they do, that's the key to success, I believe.

Friend: Yes, it is.

Me: I told my mom that for every job I had, I
loved what I was doing. I never had a job I
hated, and she said that I was lucky because
she hated every job she worked. I felt so
sorry for her. That's not a way to live. I
know back then, they had to do things they
didn't like to put food on the table

Friend: Yes, they did.

Me: I guess I should be thankful for what she
sacrificed for me and my siblings.

Friend: Yes, you should. It was tough back then.

Me: Every day I tell my mom that I love her, and
it truly comes from my heart.

Friend: Good for you. You should.


I told my friend how well my mom did on the train and in
Glenwood Springs. He was glad to hear it.

I thought the trip to Glenwood Springs would help my mom
distinguish between being on vacation and being at home. My mom
still wanted me to call her a cab to go home the day after we had
returned to FalconView. Every day, when the sun started to go down,
my mom would say she needed a ride home. I would tell her that
she was already at home. She would ask, "What city am I in?" I
answered, "You are in Colorado Springs." She would then reply, "I
don't live in Colorado."

It took me a while before I realized what was happening. My
move to Colorado Springs was not meant to be permanent.

A few days later, I was startled by a shadow standing in my
doorway at 4:00 a.m. It was Mom. I asked if anything was wrong.
She said that the people whose house we are living in had called the
police on us. She said we needed to get out of the apartment before
the police came and took us to jail. I told Mom she could stay in my
room with me, and I will take care of everything when I get up. I
turned the TV on so she could watch *The Golden Girls*. That televi-

sion show always seemed to calm her. I then tried to fall back to sleep but couldn't. I got up and made coffee.

Later that week, I developed a rash on my back. At first, my sister and I thought it was an insect bite. A few days later, it had spread over one-half of my back. There was an intense burning sensation. I went to see my nurse practitioner. The minute she looked at it, she knew it was the shingles. She gave me something to take for the pain. It didn't help. My back felt as if it was on fire. I was in so much pain. I have had broken bones and ribs, but I never felt pain as intense as this. The pain was constant. I would struggle to go to sleep at night. When I finally fell asleep, the pain would wake me right back up. Between the shingles and Mom, I was averaging four hours of sleep per night. I wondered how much sleep a person needed in order to function properly during the day. My husband used to tell me that I was the only person he knew who needed at least ten hours of sleep per night. I was in my thirties then. I am now in my sixties. According to a CDC article, people between sixty-one and sixty-four years of age need seven to nine hours of sleep per night. The article read:

> Getting enough sleep is important for people of all ages to stay in good health. People often cut back on their sleep for work, for family demands, or even to watch a good show on television. But if not getting enough sleep is a regular part of your routine, you may be at an increased risk for obesity, type 2 diabetes, high blood pressure, heart disease and stroke, poor mental health, and even early death. Even one night of short sleep can affect you the next day. Not only are you more likely to feel sleepy, but you're more likely to be in a bad mood and be less productive in your daily activities.

Neither my mother nor I was getting the recommended amount of sleep per night. This could explain our mood. This could also explain why Mom wanted us to keep the shades down in our apartment, or maybe not. Mom kept the shades down because she kept seeing people standing outside and looking in our apartment. I don't see how that was possible seeing that the apartment is on the second floor. She didn't realize how much my sister and I enjoyed looking at the panoramic view of the Rockies. Mom had turned our apartment with scenic views into a cave. That was our cue for the final phase of our life. We knew we had to take Mom back home to St. Louis, but how on earth were we going to get out of an eighteen-month lease only four months in?

Well, we didn't know the answer, but God did!

The previous Friday, a mysterious package had been delivered to our apartment. Mom had received the package from the courier, which was out of the ordinary in itself. Not knowing how to operate the chairlift we had installed for her; she made her way down and back up a flight of stairs with eighteen steps. We were so thankful to God that she didn't fall. The package was addressed to someone we did not recognize; however, it was correctly forwarded from our old address at Affinity to our new address at FalconView. Anyway, the FalconView office had closed for the day, so my sister decided she would deal with it on Monday.

Monday morning came, and my sister was planning to drop the package by the office on her way to do errands. Mom commented on how spiffy she looked to just be running errands. We thought nothing of it at the time.

When my sister arrived at the FalconView office, both of the ladies that normally worked the front office appeared to be busy, and someone, whom my sister had never met, appeared from the back office. The woman introduced herself as the manager. My sister introduced herself and told her why she was there. After handing her the package and turning to walk out the door, the woman asked, "Aren't you in the apartment that installed the chairlift?"

"Yes," my sister replied, "and if you have a minute, I'd like to talk to you about that." She did have a minute, and my sister began to explain that once our lease was up, we were planning to take Mom, who suffers from Alzheimer's disease, back home to St. Louis so that she would be in familiar surroundings, and we would be near family members to help take care of her, and we were wondering if we could donate the chairlift to the apartment complex.

As it turned out, the manager's Mom also suffered from dementia. After a lengthy conversation, the manager suggested that my sister submit a hardship request to the owners of the apartment complex to get out of the lease early. My sister called me after she left the FalconView office before she continued with the remaining errands. We both felt this was a gift from God and agreed we'd pray about it.

In the meantime, as my sister was out finishing up the remainder of her errands, Mom decided that she was really going home and proceeded down the stairs *again* and out the door this time. Being disabled myself, there was no way I could run after her, so I called my sister on her cell phone to let her know what had happened. My sister was still fifteen to twenty minutes away from the apartment, so she called the FalconView office and spoke to the woman she had just met to ask for help.

The FalconView manager was more than willing to help and walked over to the apartment to make sure everything was okay. By then, Mom had returned, and this story had a happy ending; but what about next time? My sister and I knew then that we had to move and move soon.

We spent the week drafting the hardship letter. The words flowed easily as if the Lord himself were writing it. We finished and submitted the letter that Friday and had approval that following Monday! In sixty days, we would be moving Mom back home to St. Louis. When God moves, it's mighty and awesome and powerful!

We now look back on that day my sister dropped the mysterious package off at the FalconView office and met someone that normally doesn't work the front office, who just happened to have a mom who also suffers from dementia and realize that my sister did not get all spiffed up just to run errands, but indeed she had a divine appointment!

My sister invited a few of her friends in Colorado to FalconView for a farewell dinner. We were moving Mom back to St. Louis.

It was a nice day to have our farewell dinner outside. There was a small picnic area in our apartment complex. My sister's friend put a beautiful tablecloth on the picnic table. She also adorned it with lights and freshly-cut flowers. It was beautiful. My sister's friends had been very welcoming to us.

I met my sister's friend Anne Mabry when we first moved to Affinity. I told her about how I felt when I had raised my voice at my mother. She told me to not be hard on myself for being human. I knew at that moment she was a good person. I felt privileged to have met her.

My sister's friends in Colorado seemed to care about her deeply. She had lived in Colorado Springs for over thirty years. We both decided that it was not about us anymore. It was about our mom and her needs. We wanted to get her back to her familiar surroundings, close to where she had lived all her life. We wanted our mom to feel like she was at home. Colorado was a vacation and not home to her.

I never saw my sister work as hard as she did in preparing for her move to St. Louis. She had to donate, store, and pack thirty years of accumulation. It was both emotional and inspirational to watch. I saw God all around her giving support and guidance.

As I watched my sister interact with her friends at her farewell dinner, I thought about how much had happened during our short time in Colorado. Losing my husband was one thing I wasn't prepared for. He never made it to FalconView. He died last July 21, 2021. Yet, I believed he preferred spending his last days in Colorado Springs instead of St. Louis, Missouri. My sister's friend Pamela, who planned the farewell picnic, asked me if I was looking forward to going back to St. Louis. I responded in tears. It had hit me that I was a widow. I was going back without my husband. I wiped the tears from my face as I said, "I feel sad because this move will be without my husband. I feel relieved because my sister is coming with me. And I feel confident that my sister and I have made the right decision to take our mom back home to be near her family and friends."

Hopefully, this will be Mom's final move as we pull the shades down for good on FalconView!

# CHAPTER 8

# Our Final Destination

The date was October 1, 2021.

The time was 6:00 a.m.

My alarm clock went off.

We got dressed, packed the car, and left Colorado Springs headed to our final destination, back to my daughter's house on Pyrenees Drive!

This was the seventh time within the last five years that I have packed up my mom and moved. I recently read that moving is hard on people with Alzheimer's. These moves hadn't been easy on Mom. It was probably why she could never get out of vacation mode.

I remembered our first night at Affinity, Mom wouldn't sleep in her bedroom by herself. I had to sleep with her. The same thing happened when we moved to Falcon View. I didn't know if she would react the same when we return to St. Louis. I hoped these moves have not made my mom's condition worse. I believed all these moves were necessary. We would all finally be under one roof. My mom, daughter, sister, and me. It took several years and several moves to get where we needed to be.

We would stop in Hays for the night. It was the halfway point.

We were just about an hour from reaching our halfway point when the gas light came on. According to the computer gauge, we had enough gas to go eighty miles. Hays was seventy-five miles away. My sister and I decided to wait until we got to Hays to get gas. We drove thirty miles down the highway before we looked at the computer gauge again. We had enough gas to go fifty miles. According to the sign we just passed on the highway, we were forty-seven miles from Hays.

My sister started driving faster. I told her it didn't matter how fast we went; the gas is going to end once the mileage is up. It won't matter if we arrived in ten minutes or thirty minutes. We both laughed. I told her she was acting like Rose on *The Golden Girls*. She was supposed to be more like Dorothy who was the smartest. We both laughed again. Mom, who was sitting in the back seat, was quiet as a mouse. I wondered if she knew she was going home. I wondered if she would even be able to recognize home when she saw it.

We looked at the gas gauge ten minutes later when we passed the sign on the highway that showed Hays was forty miles away. We had enough gas to go only thirty-seven miles. We decided to stop at the next gas station to fill up. We came to an exit with a gas station right off the highway. We were going too fast to pull onto the exit once we saw the station. My sister wanted to get off the next exit and go back, but I assured her that we would pass another gas station soon.

Five miles later, we passed the sign on the highway that showed Hays was thirty-five miles away. It seemed like Hays kept getting father away. The computer gauge now showed we had enough gas to go thirty miles. We drove another five miles before we reached an exit with a gas station in sight. Hayes was now thirty miles away. We got back on the highway with a full tank. The car was full, but our stomachs were empty. We didn't want to eat until we were in Hays. It was 9:00 p.m. We were hoping the restaurants won't close before 10 p.m. We were so close, yet it felt so far away. We had gone about ten miles when flashing lights got behind us. We were being pulled over by the police.

The officer asked where we were headed. We told him that it was to Hays for the night. He asked why we were going to Hays. We told him that we had hotel reservations for the night. The officer then asked where we were going after Hays. We told him that we were going to St. Louis, Missouri. Mom was very quiet in the back seat. It could have been that she was sleepy. I was pleased that she didn't say anything to the officer. He told us that he had clocked us going ninety miles per hour. He only gave us a warning. We got back on the highway with about twenty miles left for Hayes. It was now the longest twenty miles ever. It felt like it took us an hour to go twenty miles. My sister stayed under the speed limit. When we finally arrived, we had Wendy's and then went to bed. It had been an interesting journey so far. Both my sister and I hoped that this wasn't a sample of more to come ahead.

We arrived in St. Louis at 6:00 p.m. the following day. I walked back into the beautiful home my daughter Eve and I had worked so hard to get. The home was as beautiful as I remembered. We were now living with my daughter.

I remembered about ten years ago when Mom was watching *The Golden Girls*, her favorite television sitcom. We told her that one day, we would be just like them. I called us "The Golden Girls of Color."

Mom would be Dorothy's mother, Sofia. I would be Rose without the nice rack. My sister, who is very smart, would be Dorothy. My daughter Christie would be Blanche, who always acted like the youngest of the group.

We had officially moved all our things into Eve's home on October 15. The holidays were approaching. Mom's and my eating habits had changed for the better during the year and a half we spent in Colorado. My sister enjoyed cooking. We ate more home-cooked meals instead of fast food. It showed in our weight and health. We had more energy and less aches and pains. I needed the home-cooked meals to continue in St. Louis.

My sister and daughter were planning the dinner menu for the upcoming holidays. They decided that we were not celebrating Thanksgiving and Christmas this year because we considered them pagan holidays. No one knew when Jesus was born. We agreed we should be thankful more than once a year. We were going to have a family dinner on Friday after Thanksgiving. My sister was going to cook. We were going to have a rack of lamb for the first time.

The next big family feast would be on my daughter's birthday, which is December 24. My daughter Eve would cook that meal.

Mom's youngest son, Kevin, and his girlfriend were going to spend Thanksgiving with us. Mom hadn't seen her son in a couple of years or more. We found out that his girlfriend, Heather, was recently hit by a car as she was crossing the street. Her leg was in a cast. My brother had left his last place of employment to care for her. My sister and I thought it would be nice for them to stay with us for a couple of days. It was always good to be with family, especially during difficult times.

Friday's dinner was very good. The family sat in the dining room together around the table. My brother Kevin said the blessing. Everyone enjoyed eating a rack of lamb for the first time. I was the only one who ate it rare. My sister had to put everyone else's portion back into the oven until it was no longer pink on the inside. My family never learned how to eat meat correctly. If it didn't eat like shoe leather, it wasn't meat to them. LOL.

The conversation at the table centered on childhood memories. My little brother remembered when he fed all the children in the neighborhood by throwing bread and bologna out of the upstairs bedroom window in our apartment. We lived in what was once considered upscale government housing. My stepdad, Jake, got the three-bedroom apartment for us just before Kevin was born. We moved from a one-bedroom to a three-bedroom apartment. Jake died a year later. There was Mom, my sister, my two brothers, and me. I was the oldest, which put me in charge when Mom was at work. My little brother always made friends wherever we went. He had a personality and smile that drew people in. I always believed his personality would take him far in life. I never understood why his biggest dream as a child was to grow up and drive a garbage truck. Kevin would pick up anything around the house and pretend it was a steering wheel. His favorite was a vinyl record because it was round. He would make sounds to resemble a motor and lean to the side as he turned corners. He would sometimes use a clothes hanger or a stick as his steering wheel when he couldn't find a 45 vinyl record. I would laugh every time I saw him in action. His little feet moved fast and stopped on a dime when he came to an imaginary stop light. Then when the light turned green, he would take off again as his little squeaky voice reveled up his engine.

I asked my brother at the dinner table if he still wanted to drive a garbage truck. Kevin would be forty-nine next month. His birthday is on January 11. I really enjoyed his company at the dinner table. This would not have been possible if we were still in Colorado. We would not have been able to add such a memory to our precious memory bank. I watched as my brother spent time with his mom. He was so attentive to her. She enjoyed his sense of humor, his smile, and his hugs. She may not remember them tomorrow, but I will, and I will tell her about it every chance I get.

The time was 8:00 a.m.

My cell phone buzzed.

I went into Mom's room which was next to mine. She was already up. I gave Mom her medication. I then helped her get cleaned and dressed.

Today, I was taking my family to Pere Marquette Lodge for lunch.

This was a special place for me. My late husband, David, and I ate lunch at the lodge many times. Most of our day trips involved spending time at Pere Marquette Lodge. We would bring a book to read and spend the whole day sitting in the beautiful lobby with high beamed ceilings and a huge woodburning fireplace.

One time, David and I spent a night at the hotel in Pere Marquette. It was a night I would never forget because I almost died. My husband and I went swimming in their indoor pool that evening. I had taken private swimming lessons at the YMCA where I learned how to float. David and I were the only ones in the swimming pool. Later, we moved from the pool to the Jacuzzi. He turned on the bubbles. I laid my head back, shut my eyes, and never knew when my husband left the room. Twenty minutes later, the bubbles stopped. I felt my feet going up and my head going down into the water. I thought someone was pushing me under. I couldn't raise myself up. I struggled to get on my feet. I tried to yell for my husband. I tried to yell for help. I kept trying to raise my head above the water, but I couldn't. I didn't have the strength to raise myself up in the Jacuzzi. I started gasping for air. Suddenly, I felt someone lift me onto my feet. I opened my eyes, and there was a stranger standing beside me. I thanked him. I then looked for my husband. He was nowhere to be seen. I just stood up in the Jacuzzi hoping he would come back soon. I was very upset with him for leaving me.

Minutes later, he returned. I told him what had happened. He said he had just stepped out for a quick smoke and couldn't get back in the door he had gone out of, so he had to walk around to the front of the building. I told him that his smoking would be the death of me. He then helped me out of the Jacuzzi, and we went to our hotel room. I thought about how silly he would have looked if he had returned and found that I had drowned. I hoped that he would have felt guilty the rest of his life, and I would haunt him until he couldn't take it any longer.

I decided not to share that experience with my family as we drove to Pere Marquette that day. Instead, I told them David and I always enjoyed the food at their restaurant.

It was cloudy and rainy. It wasn't the perfect day for a road trip. I had no control over the weather, but I was determined to have some control over our mood. We stopped and ordered Krispy Kreme donuts to enjoy on the road. The drive was very scenic. There was the Mississippi River on one side of the road and tall cliffs on the other side. We ate Krispy Kreme donuts and listened to spiritual music. I named our road trip "Sweet Jesus!" The drive was forty-five minutes of pure bliss. I told my sister that we, golden girls of color, knew how to travel.

We pulled up in front of the Pere Marquette Lodge in Grafton, Illinois. My mom didn't want to get out of the car because it was rainy, and she was cold. She said if she got wet, she would catch a cold. My daughter went in to check things out. She came out looking very excited. She said it was so beautiful inside.

We decided, since Mom didn't want to get out, and we weren't ready to have lunch, we would take a drive around the area. I showed them the scenic path David and I used to take. The secluded road took us high above the lodge. It overlooked the river and the valley below. My daughter pulled over to get out and take pictures. We pulled up near a parked car that had steamy windows. Once my daughter realized there were people inside the car, she immediately got back inside our car and drove farther down the road to take pictures. Twenty minutes later, we returned to the lodge. The rain stopped. Mom got out and went inside with us. She admired the huge Christmas tree in the lobby. The lobby was just as I remembered, very roomy and beautiful. It still had the life-size chess set on the floor in the lobby. We went to the restaurant. Mom and I ordered the family-style fried chicken. My daughter and sister ordered the veggie burger. Everyone enjoyed their meal. It was a pleasure to see Mom enjoy the fried chicken.

My sister and daughter said we shouldn't take Mom on trips like this because she always complained. I disagreed with them. I knew they meant well. They don't like seeing our mom miserable. They believed that every time Mom complained, it was because she was miserable. I have lived with Mom longer than anyone. I knew how to take in the context of her complaining. When she wanted to be a part of our conversation, she would say something to get our affection. It didn't mean that she wanted to go home or stop doing whatever it was we were doing. My sister and daughter don't realize that how Mom felt now would be different five minutes later. It didn't matter if she was at home or out on a day trip. Mom was cold at 9 a.m. She wasn't cold at 9:30 a.m. Mom didn't want to get out of the car at 10:00 a.m. because she really wasn't hungry, though she said her back was hurting. Thirty minutes later, when Mom was ready to eat lunch, she was able to get out of the car and walk to the restaurant. She never complained. In the restaurant, Mom was cold. Her mood seemed low. She complained about how uncomfortable the chairs were. She complained about how hard the bread was. She complained about not having any money to pay for her food. When the food came and everyone started eating, Mom's complaining ceased. She stopped worrying about not being able to pay for her food. She didn't even seem to mind how hard the chairs were or how cold she was. Her frown always ended upside down. She complained at home as well as out, so why not take her out so she can enjoy good food in the company of her loved ones? The day trip ended as I knew it would—on a good note. That's why I put myself in charge of Mom's entertainment and my sister in charge of Mom's nutrition and my daughter in charge of Mom's hygiene.

I'm not saying I will always know what's best for Mom. I have made mistakes and will probably make more mistakes. I don't pretend to be an expert on how to care for a loved one with dementia. I just know how to have fun with the lady I knew before she had dementia.

I planned a longer outing with Mom after my daughter's birthday. My daughter, Eve, will be turning forty-five years old. My sister was baking Eve's favorite strawberry cake. My daughter was going to cook her children's favorite dishes—baked macaroni, chicken and dressing, sweet potatoes, along with something different—Eve wanted my sister to make the rack of lamb again.

My grandchildren were going to spend the night here on their mother's birthday. It had been a tradition for the past four or five years. My sister, who had lived alone most of her life, had planned to spend the night at a hotel. She was not used to being around many people during the holidays. She had lived by herself in Colorado for over thirty years. This was new to her. My daughter and I understood that she needed her privacy. We respected her wishes.

On December 24, at midnight, I wanted to be the first to wish my daughter a happy birthday. I let her open her birthday card. I then went to bed so I could be awake for Mom who gets up at 4:00 or 5:00 a.m. I was responsible for her taking her medicine an hour before breakfast.

My grandchildren planned to arrive at 6:00 p.m. We planned to have dinner at 7:00 p.m. Everyone started arriving closer to 6:30 p.m. My youngest grandson KenKen was the first to arrive. He came in the house bearing gifts. He reminded me of myself during this time of the year. I used to take the holidays very seriously. I brought gifts for everyone. I couldn't wait to see the expression on my family's faces as they opened their gifts. It was my joy. I spent the whole year preparing for this one evening. I tried to make sure my grandchildren got what they asked for. The boys were into video games. I always tried to get the latest one for them. My granddaughter was always a fashionista.

Last year, I was in Colorado, so I didn't participate in the family event. This year, I was here with my family, but I had stopped celebrating Christmas. This year was the hardest for me. My husband died a few months ago, my mother's Alzheimer's had gotten much worse, and I won't be participating with my grandchildren on Christmas. I felt like Scrooge.

I enjoyed eating dinner at the table with my grandchildren. I listened to them talk about what activities they had been involved in the previous year. They talked about their successes and their disappointments. It was nice catching up with my grandchildren. After dinner, we went downstairs to watch my great grandchildren open their gifts. I was surprised when I was given gifts to open. I wasn't expecting gifts. It was a pleasant surprise. I will make up for it on their birthdays.

I always enjoyed watching my daughter interact with her children and grandchildren. She seemed happy on her birthday being surrounded by family. Unfortunately, the noise and commotion were a little too much for my mom. She couldn't seem to understand what was happening, which always irritated her. We were able to get her to calm down once my grandson handed her a handful of lottery scratch-offs. She started scratching her tickets immediately. She had fun, although she didn't have any winners. Everyone checked Mom's lottery tickets after she did to make sure she didn't miss any winners.

December 24 at Eve's house was very jovial. The atmosphere was full of awe and laughter. It didn't matter that we no longer enjoyed Christmas because my daughter's birthday would bring enough joy into the home every year.

The date was January 12, 2022.

The time was 8:00 a.m.

My cell phone ringer went off.

I answered to find it was my customer. He may have to cancel his trip tomorrow. One of his traveling companions may be too ill to travel. He wanted to know if he would receive credit and how long would the credit be good for.

I was glad to receive the call, although I wish it had been under better circumstances. I needed to get up to start packing for Mom and my little trip to Lake of the Ozarks. It's the four "Golden Girls of Color" heading out for more adventure.

I wanted to leave at noon, but we didn't get on the road until 3:00 p.m. My sister had to take care of a Shaklee order that took longer than she had expected. My daughter had to take care of a customer who wanted to pay for their upcoming cruise. I had to call in an Amtrak Vacations reservation for a guest. We were all working three hours longer than we planned.

We finally packed the car and got on the road. We had a three-hour drive. We would arrive at the hotel just in time for dinner at 7:00 p.m.

It had gotten dark outside before we arrived at the hotel. I was looking forward to seeing the view outside the window in our junior suite. Unfortunately, I had to wait till morning. I liked the size of the suite. We had a sitting area with a sleeper sofa. There was a desk area by the window to work at. There was also a kitchenette with a sink and counter to sit at to eat. It was roomy for four adults. My sister was impressed with the bathroom, although there wasn't a bathtub for her to soak in.

My daughter, Eve, and my sister went downstairs to the bar to order dinner. They came back to the room with a grilled chicken sandwich, chicken wings, turkey wrap, and french fries. The bar food wasn't that great. Mom had gone to bed before the food arrived. She looked at it and wasn't impressed enough to get up and eat her dinner. She told Eve to put it in the fridge, and she would have it for breakfast.

The following morning, I was eager to get dressed and walk around the hotel. My sister joined me. We started on the lower level where the bar and indoor pool were located. There weren't many guests at the hotel, so we received personal service. A female staff member in the workout room showed us where the private massage room was located. She also told us there was a Jacuzzi in the women's locker room.

I liked the game room and bar area. It had something for everyone to do. You could sit at the bar and have a cocktail or walk over to the game room and play a game of pool, air hockey, darts, ping pong, etc.

This was my ideal hotel because I didn't need to go out for anything. I could spend a couple of days either relaxing, swimming, drinking, reading, or playing games with the family. I planned to visit often.

Later that day, my sister and my daughter took Mom and me to enjoy the recliners in the private massage room. Mom sat in one and my daughter sat in the other one beside her. There were only two massage chairs in the room. It was a great place for couples to go and relax. My mom turned on the chair, and it started moving. She started yelling. She said it felt like someone started beating her on the back. She then pushes the buttons for the feet, which caused her to start laughing hysterically. She said it was tickling her feet. Mom pushed another button that started reclining. She thought it was going to throw her over on her head. She yelled for one of us to turn the chair off. I tried to but it wouldn't go down. My mom said she was going to jump out of the chair. I begged her not to. I didn't want her to hurt herself. My sister went to look for help. In the meantime, my daughter was in the chair next to Mom, crying that she was being massaged too hard. My daughter couldn't get out of her chair either. I was laughing at the same time I was worried. Mom kept saying she was going to jump out of the chair, and I kept begging her to wait till help arrived. The expressions on both my mother's and daughter's faces every time the rollers moved up and down their backs were priceless while scary at the same time. Both looked as if the chairs were giving them electric shock treatments.

My sister arrived with a hotel staff member. He couldn't help but laugh at what he saw when we entered the room. He jokingly asked Mom how she broke his chair. He kept trying to get the chair to go down for Mom to get out, but he couldn't. It took a while for him to figure out how to get Mom out of the chair. I don't know if Mom will ever sit in a massage chair again. We then took her out into the game room to play air hockey. She remembered that she used to play it and how much she enjoyed it. After a couple of hours in the game room and a couple of margaritas for me, we went upstairs to the Royal Restaurant for dinner.

This was right after New Year's. We were the only ones in the restaurant. My sister took pictures of the elegant decor. My mother, sister, daughter, and I sat at dinner talking about our day.

This short vacation seemed perfect for Mom. It wasn't overwhelming as the cruises had been. There wasn't much of a crowd. There wasn't much noise. The drive here was only three hours. The hotel had just enough things to do without having to go out. I was so impressed with how much walking Mom had done. She did complain about her back, but she didn't let it slow her down. Mom's famous words were "Use it before you lose it."

We checked out of the hotel the following day. During our drive home, Mom said the same thing she did when I took her to Glenwood Springs for a three-day vacation. It's the one thing that always lets me know how important these trips are—"This was a nice vacation!" Those five little words let me know that Mom was still having fun! I won't stop till she stops, which I pray will be a very long time from now!

I know not everyone is able to be a caregiver. But everyone has the heart to make sure their loved ones get the care they need. And when the time comes to say goodbye, you are at peace knowing their time had been well spent!

www.ingramcontent.com/pod-product-compliance
Lightning Source LLC
Chambersburg PA
CBHW022050150726
47990CB00003B/1034